MEDICAL BILLING AND CODING FOR BEGINNERS

By

Sean D. Carlson

TABLE OF CONTENTS

#1 Medical Billing & Coding

#2 CPC EXAM

#3 Medical Terminology

INTRODUCTION: THE POTENTIAL OF MEDICAL BILLING AND CODING

> Medical billing and coding jobs are on the rise and expected to grow at 8% through 2029. This is double the national average job growth.
>
> —U.S. Bureau of Labor Statistics

The Unique Benefits of a Career in Medical Billing and Coding

There are several benefits attached to having a career in medical billing and coding, and they include:

Getting a rewarding career in health care

There's no need to work directly in patient care to enjoy a rewarding career in health care. As a medical biller and coder, you will ensure that healthcare providers receive adequate compensation for the care offered and help patients get the maximum benefit from their insurance.

Working in different settings, including your home

Hospitals, doctors' offices, and insurance agencies are the most common medical billing and coding job settings. Government agencies also employ medical billers and coders, as do the National Center for Health Statistics and Medicaid offices. Some medical billing and coding professionals are staff of companies that develop medical software, while others are staff of educational institutions that train other medical billers and coders. There's also the option to work from your own home.

Earning a good salary

According to the U.S. Bureau of Labor Statistics (BLS), the median annual wage for medical records specialists (which includes medical billers and coders) was $48,780 in May 2024. While this figure reflects the median, there is certainly room for earning more with certifications. The AAPC 2024 Salary Survey found that certified coders earn an average of $59,895 annually, a significant 22.8% more than their non-certified counterparts. Moreover, the survey confirms that obtaining multiple certifications can further boost your salary potential, leading to even higher earnings in the field.

Enjoying predictable work hours

Most healthcare careers want you to be on call and work during weekends, holidays, and every hour of the day. That's not the same for medical billing and coding jobs. You have a predictable schedule, and there's room for working remotely as a medical biller and coder.

Increasing demand for medical billers and coders

Medical billing and coding jobs are rising and should grow approximately 8% through 2029. The BLS stated that this is twice the national average job growth rate, and it predicts that there will be an additional 15,000 new medical billing and coding jobs annually for the next eight years.

Having job stability during an economic downturn

The demand for experienced medical billers and coders will keep rising. Therefore, employment in this field will increase as the population in the United States ages. An aging population indicates that there will be an increase in claims submitted for reimbursement from insurance companies as more medical care is offered.

Working in your new career within a year

This healthcare career doesn't require you to spend years in school. There are opportunities to complete professional medical billing and coding courses online in a year and start working in your new career instantly thereafter. You can also earn a highly recognized medical billing and coding certification to prove your skills further and increase your opportunities to increase your salary.

Offering an essential service as a member of the healthcare team

As a medical biller and coder, you will assign the right codes to patient diagnoses and then request payment from insurance companies. This profession enables healthcare providers to receive the correct payment for the treatment offered. Most of your time will involve sitting in front of a computer while organizing statements, reviewing bills, assigning codes, and performing quality control. You should also be detail-oriented and willing to collaborate with others for accuracy in the work.

Enjoying opportunities for advancement

Many paths can help you advance your healthcare career when you become a medical biller and coder. After gaining experience, consider a supervisory role as a billing or coding supervisor or a medical or health services manager. Furthermore, you could also become a medical biller and coder and assist people with your knowledge of medical terminology and the healthcare system. Then you can return to school to earn a degree in data management, nursing, or even pre-med.

Short Personal Story of the Author: How I Discovered Medical Billing and Coding—My Journey to Becoming a Professional and the Benefits I've Personally Experienced

Medical billing and coding is a great career path with a promising and fulfilling experience for anyone in the healthcare industry. As a writer and advocate for this field, I can attest to the fact that people who seek a profession that blends their passion for healthcare with organizational skills and attention to detail have come to the right place.

During my high school years, I was a volunteer at a local hospital where I observed the committed professionals who work behind the scenes for healthcare providers to receive the proper compensation. So I was inspired to explore the world of medical billing and coding and later realized that I loved it.

This is why I wrote this detailed book: *Medical Billing and Coding for Beginners*. I want to guide aspiring professionals with all the necessary information to thrive in the field.

I had to immerse myself in the world of medical terminology, coding systems, insurance processes, and regulatory guidelines so that this book became the solid groundwork for readers who want to prepare for certification exams and enhance their professional credentials. Every chapter that I wrote assured me that unlimited opportunities lay ahead.

The people who embraced this career path after reading my book gave testimonies. One of them includes realizing their key role in the healthcare sector. They could accurately assign codes and process insurance claims for healthcare providers to ensure they were properly compensated and were able to contribute to the industry's overall functioning.

They were also grateful for the flexibility of this career by working in various settings, including hospitals, doctors' offices, insurance agencies, and remotely. This flexibility further indicates that this career supports a work-life balance for anyone to pursue personal interests and enjoy quality time with their loved ones.

Let's not forget the financial aspects of the profession. The salary is competitive and includes options for additional certifications and experience to boost your earnings. Therefore, there is financial stability and an opportunity for personal growth and advancement in this aspect of the healthcare industry.

I also noted that these professionals have been honing their skills and engaging in continual learning to cope with the demands of this evolving field. This book still helped them explore opportunities for growth and advancement that allowed them to gain supervisory roles, higher education in related fields, and even leadership positions.

Once again, the world of medical billing and coding has been a great experience, and writing this impactful book was worthwhile.

My story shows that anyone with curiosity and exploration can find fulfilling paths.

Therefore, trust the information in this book to guide you as you prepare for this career. I've broken complex subjects down into simpler terms. My experiences helped me create practical tips, real-world examples, and valuable insights you will enjoy. Just follow the guidance provided to help you easily maneuver industry challenges and achieve your career goals.

Since skilled medical billing and coding professionals will always be in demand in the industry, I will keep improving and expanding the available resources, such as creating online courses and workshops and writing additional books that focus on diverse skill levels and specialized areas within the field so that an aspiring medical biller and coder can access the required tools and knowledge for success.

In summary, my journey from curiosity to writing this book has been transformative because sharing my knowledge and experiences has empowered others to obtain an appealing career path in medical billing and coding.

GET YOUR BONUSES

Don't forget to download your free bonuses! Go to the last page of the book. Enjoy your reading!

CHAPTER 1: EXPLORING MEDICAL BILLING AND CODING

I love that this field means you can contribute to the
healthcare industry if you don't like blood and guts
but are still interested in the medical field.

—Robyn Korn, MBA, RHIA, CPHQ, Adjunct
Instructor of Medical Coding at Purdue University Global

This chapter will define medical billing and coding in ways that will allow you to understand its complexities. Then, we'll discuss the key roles and responsibilities of a medical biller and coder. The last section will focus on the structure and significance of medical codes. And now, let's begin!

Detailed Explanation of What Medical Billing and Coding Is

What Is Medical Billing?

You can also refer to medical coding as medical classification, and it's also similar to translation. Medical coding is converting health information and patient data (e.g., the diagnosis, procedures, medical services, and equipment) into a universal medical alphanumeric code. You can collect data from patient records, physician's notes, lab results, and other documentation and translate it into a code that insurance companies can decode. Therefore, before any diagnosis and medical procedure, there must be a corresponding medical code.

What Is Medical Coding?

Medical coding is when you translate health information and patient data, such as diagnoses, procedures, medical services, and equipment used, into universal alphanumeric codes that can be obtained from various sources like patient records, physician's notes, and lab results. These codes allow insurance companies to decode the available information easily.

Note that there are many codes in medical coding, and each corresponds to a certain procedure, service, illness, or injury.

For clinicians, medical facilities, insurance companies, government agencies, and other healthcare organizations, these codes are a universal language. You can create these codes through specific coding classification systems like CPT®, ICD-10-CM, and HCPCS Level II.

After accurately determining and verifying these codes as a medical biller and coder, you enter them into a system and transfer them to the medical biller. Accurate coding boosts precise billing for healthcare providers for efficient financial operations.

What Is Medical Billing and Coding?

Medical billing and coding occur when you convert patient charts and clinical data to medical claims and submit them to payers for reimbursement.

Understanding the Key Roles and Responsibilities of a Medical Biller and Coder

Medical Biller Responsibilities

The medical billing job description is as simple as creating and sending medical claims for the insurance companies and the patients.

A medical biller should report accurate information to the insurance company so the patient will be billed correctly.

Once the insurance company has paid its portion, medical billers receive the remaining bill prepared and sent to the patient.

In addition, a medical biller may follow up on unpaid claims, clarify discrepancies, organize payment plans for patients, obtain pre-authorization for certain procedures, review bills, verify eligibility, etc.

Medical Billing Job Duties

Medical billers have the following job duties:

- They validate coverage and eligibility for medical services.

- They communicate with insurance providers and patients.

- They review and correct patient bills.

- They prepare and transfer claims via billing software.

- They gather unpaid claims and handle discrepancies.

17

- They do research and appeal denied claims.

- They update spreadsheets and reports via data entry.

- They assist patients in creating payment plans.

- They exhibit flexibility to changes in the billing software.

Medical Coder Responsibilities

A medical coder should assist the healthcare system in securing payments from insurance providers for medical services such as office visits, routine exams, advanced procedures, etc.

Typical job descriptions involve reviewing patient information, converting that information into universal medical codes, and completing data entry to submit forms and claim details to the medical biller.

Medical Coding Job Duties

Medical coders have the following job duties:

- They review patient information and translate services into proper codes.

- They enter medical data into patient account systems.

- They complete different given tasks per day.

- They are familiar with universal code classifications like the International Classification of Diseases (ICD-10) and Current Procedural Terminology (CPT).

- They communicate with insurance providers and medical staff.

The Structure and Significance of Medical Codes

The healthcare system employs medical codes to achieve a structured and standardized format for classifying and communicating information related to medical diagnoses, procedures, treatments, and services. The two main coding systems in this profession are the ICD and CPT systems.

The ICD code can be used to document and categorize diseases, injuries, symptoms, and other health conditions. In 2019, the WHO produced its 11th revision, ICD-11, of the International Classification of Diseases, which is a globally accepted standard for medical coding and classification. ICD-11 was released on January 1, 2022, to provide a clear and flexible framework for organizing diseases, injuries, and health-related conditions. It also follows a chapter-based structure along with various body systems and assigns alphanumeric codes to individual conditions or groups of related conditions. If you want more information, refer to the latest version of ICD-11.

On the other hand, CPT codes can be used to identify medical procedures, treatments, and services performed by healthcare providers. With these codes, you can get a standardized approach to describe and bill healthcare services for accurate communication and reimbursement processes.

Key Takeaways:

- Medical billing is when you convert health information and patient data (e.g., the diagnosis, procedures, medical services, and equipment used) into a universal medical alphanumeric code. Medical coding occurs when you translate health information and patient data, like diagnoses, procedures, medical services, and equipment used, into universal alphanumeric codes.

- Medical codes like the ICD and CPT provide a structured, standardized method to classify and communicate medical information.

- Medical billers should create and submit claims, follow up on unpaid claims, and coordinate payment plans with patients.

- Medical coders should review patient information and translate it into proper codes for accurate reimbursement.

- Medical codes can be used to bill, reimburse, analyze data, improve quality, support clinical decisions, and plan for healthcare.

Next, you will gain a deeper understanding of medical coding systems. Check out the next chapter to learn more about these essential systems.

CHAPTER 2: DIVING INTO MEDICAL CODING SYSTEMS

This chapter focuses on the fundamental coding systems used in the medical field. Now, you will thoroughly understand these terms: International Classification of Diseases (ICD), Current Procedural Terminology (CPT), Healthcare Common Procedure Coding System (HCPCS), Systematized Nomenclature of Medicine–Clinical Terms (SNOMED CT), and Logical Observation Identifiers Names and Codes (LOINC).

Understanding the International Classification of Diseases (ICD)

What Is the International Classification of Diseases (ICD)?

The ICD is a diagnostic tool used worldwide for epidemiology, health management, and clinical purposes. The ICD is managed by the WHO as the director and coordinator for health within the United Nations System. This tool was mainly developed as a healthcare classification method that offers a system of diagnostic codes to classify diseases, such as nuanced classifications of several signs, symptoms, abnormal findings, complaints, social circumstances, and external causes of injury or disease. This system's purpose is to map health conditions to corresponding generic categories as well as specific variations, assigning for these a designated code of up to six characters in length. As a result, major categories are created to have a set of similar diseases.

The WHO made the ICD available globally for various purposes, such as morbidity and mortality statistics, reimbursement systems, and automated decision support in health care. The ICD enables international comparability in the collection, processing, classification, and presentation of these statistics.

This means that the ICD is a major program used to classify all health disorders statistically, providing diagnostic assistance and serving as the main statistically-based classificatory diagnostic system for healthcare-related issues for the WHO Family of International Classifications (WHO-FIC).

Also, note that the ICD is revised periodically and is now in its 11th revision. As mentioned in the previous chapter, on May 25, 2019, the WHO's World Health Assembly (WHA) adopted the ICD-11 and introduced it on January 1, 2022. Then, on February 11, 2022, the WHO announced that 35 countries were using the ICD-11.

The ICD belongs to a "family" of international classifications (WHO-FIC) that complement each other, including the International Classification of Functioning, Disability, and Health (ICF). They all focus on the domains of functioning (disability) related to health conditions from both medical and social perspectives. Also, the International Classification of Health Interventions (ICHI) plays an important role in classifying all medical, nursing, functioning, and public health interventions.

The formal title of the ICD is the International Statistical Classification of Diseases and Related Health Problems; nevertheless, the original title, International Classification of Diseases, is still its generic name.

Note that the United States and some other countries use the Diagnostic and Statistical Manual of Mental Disorders (DSM) to classify mental disorders for some purposes.

Mental Health Issues

The ICD has a section for the classification of mental and behavioral disorders (Chapter V). This was developed with the DSM of the American Psychiatric Association, and the two manuals use similar classifications. The WHO is revising its classifications in these sections in the development of the ICD-11, and an international advisory group has been implemented to guide this.

One area of particular focus is Section F66 of the ICD-10, which addresses the classification of psychological and behavioral disorders concerning sexual development and orientation. It states that "sexual orientation by itself is not to be considered a disorder"; in addition, the DSM and other classifications identify homosexuality as a regular variation in human sexuality. The advisory group has stated that there is "no evidence that [these classifications] are clinically useful" and recommended that section F66 be removed from the ICD-11.

Additionally, an international survey of psychiatrists in 66 countries who compared the use of the ICD-10 and DSM-IV realized that the former was often used for clinical diagnosis while the latter was only for research. The ICD is the official system for classifying mental disorders internationally, yet because of the DSM's prominence, most mental health professionals in the United States mainly use the DSM.

ICD Purpose and Uses

As a classification and terminology system, ICD-11:

- Gives room to the systematic recording, analysis, interpretation, and comparison of mortality and morbidity data collected in several countries or regions and at different times.

- Enables the semantic interoperability and reusability of recorded data for the different use cases beyond regular health statistics, such as decision support, resource allocation, reimbursement guidelines, and others.

ICD-11 Highlights

- Legally accepted health data standard (WHO Constitution and Nomenclature Regulations)

- Anything occurring in January 2022

- Conceptual framework that accepts language and culture

- Integration of terminology and classification

- End-to-end digital solution (API, tools, online and offline)

- Updated scientific knowledge

- Comparable statistics and semantic interoperability for 150 years

In addition, the ICD-11 offers several advantages:

- ICD-11 is accessible.

- ICD-11 is distributed under the Creative Commons Attribution-NoDerivs 3.0 IGO license.

- ICD-11 enables the counting of traditional medicine services and encounters.

- The 11th revision of the ICD is more extensive and yields better results for any work performed with it. Unlike any revision since the 6th edition in 1948, the ICD-11 is highly productive.

Usage in the United States

In the United States, the US Public Health Service released the International Classification of Diseases, Adapted for Indexing of Hospital Records and Operation Classification (ICDA), completed in 1962, enhanced the ICD-7 in several areas to tackle the indexing needs of hospitals. After that, the US Public Health Service released the Eighth Revision, International Classification of Diseases and Adapted for Use in the United States, generally known as ICDA-8, for official national morbidity and mortality statistics.

Then we had the ICD, 9th Revision, Clinical Modification, regarded as ICD-9-CM, released by the US Department of Health and Human Services for hospitals and other healthcare facilities, which provided a better means to explain the clinical picture of the patient. The diagnosis component of ICD-9-CM fully aligns with ICD-9 codes and is still the data standard for reporting morbidity.

National adaptations of the ICD-10 advanced to add both clinical code (ICD-10-CM) and procedure code (ICD-10-PCS) with complete revisions in 2003. In 2009, the US Centers for Medicare and Medicaid Services noted that it would start using ICD-10 on April 1, 2010, with full participation by all involved parties by 2013. Yet, the US extended the deadline twice and did not formally progress to the ICD-10-CM (for most clinical encounters) until October 1, 2015.

Below are the years for the classification of the causes of death in the United States by each revision:

- ICD-1: 1900

- ICD-2: 1910

- ICD-3: 1921

- ICD-4: 1930

- ICD-5: 1939

- ICD-6: 1949

- ICD-7: 1958

- ICDA-8: 1968

- ICD-9-CM: 1979

- ICD-10-CM: 1999

The cause of death on US death certificates, statistically gathered by the Centers for Disease Control and Prevention (CDC), are coded in the ICD, which does not involve codes for human and system factors generally known as medical errors.

Exploring Current Procedural Terminology (CPT)

Current Procedural Terminology (CPT) is a medical code set for reporting medical, surgical, and diagnostic procedures and services to entities, including physicians, health insurance companies, and accreditation organizations.

How Does CPT Work?

CPT was officially introduced in 1966 and has progressed to its fifth edition. The AMA evaluates the coding every year to gauge whether a new CPT code is required. The CPT system consists of three levels of codes:

- Category I codes are the most common. They are used to report general medical procedures and services.

- Category II codes can be used to report more specific procedures and services, including those that require special training or equipment.

- Category III codes can be used for new technologies and procedures that are currently being evaluated.

Codes from all three categories can be used to bill for physician services. The AMA has developed a CPT Editorial Panel, which includes doctors from various specialties, who keep reviewing and revising the CPT code set to ensure the codes are accurately assigned to procedures.

Moreover, there is a yearly review process whereby new codes can be suggested and existing codes revised. The CPT system keeps evolving to adapt to medical technology and practice changes.

How Is the CPT Code Set Categorized?

Note that evaluation and management (E/M), surgical, and radiology services comprise the three primary CPT categories.

- E/M codes: These codes are for office visits, hospital visits, and other outpatient services; they account for the level of care offered and the time spent with the patient.

- Surgical codes: These codes cover procedures carried out in an operating room or another setting; they provide information on the procedure type, the body area involved, and the anesthesia used.

- Radiology codes: These codes identify diagnostic tests and procedures like X-rays, MRIs, and CT scans. They explain the type of test or procedure carried out and any special occurrence that may have been involved.

Ways to Find the Appropriate CPT Code(s) for the Procedure or Service You're Billing

- When billing for a healthcare procedure or service, providers should use the right CPT code (or codes) to enable insurers to reimburse them for the cost. The AMA's online CPT code database is where billers can find the correct CPT code(s).

- To search, just input key terms associated with the procedure or service. For instance, if you're billing for a skin biopsy, you might input "skin biopsy" or "biopsy, skin."

- The results usually involve a list of codes that match your search terms and a description of each code.

- After identifying the right code (or codes), go ahead and add them to your insurance claim form. Billers can ask a supervisor or another experienced medical billing professional for assistance or refer to the CPT codebook if they are unsure which codes to use.

How Can You Understand CPT Codes on a Bill?

If you're reading a medical bill, you may find CPT codes listed for the services provided. Learn what each code means to ensure accuracy and avoid errors or inconsistencies.

For example, a bill with the five-digit code "99213" indicates a type of office visit. The numbers used in the code indicate the provided level of service. A 99213, for example, is for a known patient who visited between 20–29 minutes, while a 99214 is for a known patient who visited between 30–39 minutes.

How Do Modifiers Work?

CPT modifiers are two-digit codes that give more information related to a medical service or procedure. These codes can be used to reveal a modified procedure or report a change in the normal circumstances of service.

Use the proper modifier code for accurate reimbursement when submitting claims to insurance companies. Failure to use a modifier can result in a claim denial in some cases.

There are different types of CPT modifiers, each with a specific meaning. Examples of modifiers include:

- Modifier 25: This modifier involves a separate and distinct procedure performed on the same day as another procedure.

- Modifier 50: This modifier involves a procedure performed bilaterally (on both sides).

- Modifier 51: This modifier involves a procedure carried out with multiple units.

CPT modifiers are not compulsory, yet they can often be used to ensure receipt for full reimbursement. If you have doubts, you can check with the patient's insurance company to see if a modifier is needed.

The Intricacies of the Healthcare Common Procedure Coding System (HCPCS)

The HCPCS, often known by its acronym as "hick picks," is a set of healthcare procedure codes based on the American Medical Association's Current Procedural Terminology (CPT).

History

The acronym HCPCS initially represented the HCFA Common Procedure Coding System, a medical billing process used by the Centers for Medicare and Medicaid Services (CMS). Before 2001, CMS was recognized as the Health Care Financing Administration (HCFA). In 1978, the HCPCS was founded to offer a standardized coding system for explaining the specific items and services offered in the delivery of health care.

Such coding is needed for Medicare, Medicaid, and other health insurance programs so that insurance claims can be processed in an orderly and consistent manner. At first, the use of these codes was optional; however, with the establishment of the Health Insurance Portability and Accountability Act of 1996 (HIPAA), the use of the HCPCS for transactions such as healthcare information became compulsory.

Levels of Codes

The HCPCS involves three levels of codes:

- Level I is a numeric code that includes the American Medical Association's CPT.

- Level II codes are alphanumeric and mainly involve non-physician services, such as ambulance services and prosthetic devices. These codes represent items, supplies, and nonphysician services not included in CPT-4 codes (Level I).

- Level III codes, also known as local codes, were created by state Medicaid agencies, Medicare contractors, and private insurers to use in specific programs and jurisdictions. HIPAA directed the CMS to implement a standard coding system for reporting medical transactions. However, the use of Level III codes was stopped on December 31, 2003, to comply with consistent coding standards. Level III codes were not like the modern CPT Category III codes, which were released in 2001 to code emerging technology.

Introduction to SNOMED CT (Systematized Nomenclature of Medicine – Clinical Terms)

The Systematized Nomenclature of Medicine–Clinical Terms (SNOMED CT), as a comprehensive clinical terminology system, offers a structured, detailed, and clear manner of encoding and depicting clinical concepts and terms used in health care.

As such, SNOMED CT gives meaning to clinical information.

The system has more than 350,000 unique concepts or "clinical terms" in the SNOMED CT, which is owned by the International Health Terminology Standards Development Organization (IHTSDO), also known as SNOMED International.

Use of SNOMED CT

- You can use the SNOMED CT system to record and share accurate and consistent information related to medicine, medical/clinical conditions, and health care to enhance patient care.

- Healthcare providers can use the system to communicate more effectively about a patient's condition because it provides a standardized language for explaining clinical concepts and the sharing of clinical data among systems and healthcare sectors.

- The healthcare industry can use the system for clinical decision support systems, public health reporting, research, and quality measurement to assist other healthcare-related activities, including billing, administrative reporting, and healthcare analytics.

How Can SNOMED CT Affect Healthcare?

With SNOMED CT as a universal health language, effective communication is possible among healthcare professionals, patients, and other stakeholders both within and beyond the healthcare system.

As a result, patients do not need to repeat their information when interacting with different healthcare providers, and there is improved monitoring and treatment of patients. This helps to ensure patient safety, and healthcare personnel can streamline their documentation processes to save time.

How Does SNOMED CT Work?

SNOMED CT works by arranging clinical/medical terms into a hierarchical structure of "concepts."

Concepts and Descriptions

The concepts in SNOMED CT include words and expressions used in clinical settings:

- Diseases: These are concepts for various diseases, such as pneumonia, diabetes, cancer, etc.

- Clinical findings: These are concepts for abnormal clinical findings, such as high blood pressure, abnormal heart rhythm, etc.

- Procedures: These are concepts for surgical and diagnostic procedures such as X-ray, biopsy, chemotherapy, etc.

- Anatomical structures: These are concepts for different parts of the body, such as the lungs, liver, heart, etc.

- Organisms: These are concepts for different organisms such as bacteria, viruses, etc.

- Substances: These are concepts for different substances such as drugs, chemicals, etc.

Each concept or clinical term in SNOMED CT is given a unique numerical code known as a "concept identifier" or "concept ID." This code helps to identify and obtain the clinical term in the SNOMED CT system.

Clinical terms are also given standardized names known as "fully specified names," which offer more context and a clear clarification for the term. For instance, the clinical term with the concept ID "123456789" might include the fully specified name "malignant neoplasm of the breast."

Moreover, each concept can have several synonyms. Synonyms for "malignant neoplasm of the breast" may include "breast cancer," "cancer of the breast," "mammary cancer," "invasive ductal carcinoma," and "invasive lobular carcinoma."

These synonyms may then be classified as "preferred" or "acceptable."

Relationships

Apart from its descriptions and unique numerical codes, SNOMED CT also involves relationships between concepts. These relationships determine how terms are connected to each other and can offer more context and information about a patient's medical condition.

SNOMED CT involves "is-a" relationships that connect concepts with additional general concepts higher up in the same hierarchy.

For instance, a relationship might imply that "malignant neoplasm of the breast" is a "disorder of the breast" or that "pneumonia caused by Haemophilus influenzae" is a "bacterial infectious disease."

There are also relationships that offer information concerning the features of the concept and that connect concepts from different hierarchies together.

For instance, breast cancer has an "associated morphology" with "ductal carcinoma" and an "anatomical location of finding," which is "breast." These relationships offer information concerning the disease process in the tissue and the location of the disease.

Relationships offer meaning to concepts and enable them to integrate into the extensive network of terms in SNOMED CT. Lastly, all concepts are classified as either primitive or defined. A concept is defined when its relationships can differentiate it from all other concepts in the system.

Hierarchical Structure

The SNOMED CT system organizes the concepts into a hierarchical structure. The top level includes broad categories such as "body structure" or "clinical finding," which are then subdivided into more specific subcategories.

For example, "body structure" has subcategories like "organism" and "tissue." Under "organism," we have subcategories like "human," "animal," and "bacterial." This hierarchical structure allows easy navigation and classification of clinical terms.

Concepts can be broadened or narrowed; for example, consider "injury to the knee." A broader term is "injury to the leg," whereas a narrower term is "ligament injury of the knee."

The hierarchical organization of concepts of SNOMED CT from broad to specific helps clinicians to manage information at a level of detail suitable for their needs and to be usable by various healthcare services.

This creates detailed documentation of clinical information, which can later be used and compiled at a more general level. This is why SNOMED CT improves the quality of health data and becomes more available for research and innovation.

SNOMED CT Integrations

SNOMED CT can be integrated with other broadly used coding systems like the International Classification of Primary Care (ICPC) and the ICD-10.

By being coded against these current terminologies, SNOMED CT is a vital bridge between established coding sets and allows easier implementation of standardized health language across different health services.

The integration of SNOMED CT with other code sets improves interoperability and fosters better sharing and exchange of clinical data among healthcare providers to increase services to the highest quality and safety of patient care.

Summary

SNOMED CT is growing more relevant in the healthcare industry as more organizations consider digitization and standardization of clinical information. It helps to enhance the quality and safety of patient care, promoting interoperability and better clinical decision-making.

Overview of Logical Observation Identifiers Names and Codes (LOINC)

Logical observation identifiers names and codes (LOINC) is a database and universal standard to identify medical laboratory observations. It was established in 1994 and is managed by the Regenstrief Institute, a US nonprofit medical research organization. LOINC was developed to address the demand for an electronic database for clinical care and management and is publicly available for free.

The American Clinical Laboratory Association has endorsed LOINC. Since it was introduced, the database has gone beyond just including medical laboratory code names to also incorporating nursing diagnoses, nursing interventions, outcomes classification, and patient care data sets.

Function

LOINC assigns universal code names and identifiers to medical terminology associated with electronic health records. This is done to assist in the electronic exchange and gathering of clinical results, such as laboratory tests, clinical observations, outcomes management, and research. LOINC has two main parts: laboratory LOINC and clinical LOINC. Clinical LOINC has a subdomain, Document Ontology, which captures clinical reports and documents.

Many standards like Integrating the Healthcare Enterprise (IHE) or Health Level 7 (HL7) use LOINC to electronically pass results from various reporting systems to the right healthcare networks. Healthcare professionals and the healthcare industry have adopted IHE as a way to improve the way healthcare computer systems share information with each other. With a goal of optimizing patient care, IHE promotes the coordinated use of established coding standards such as Digital Imaging and Communications in Medicine (DICOM) and HL7 to address specific clinical needs for patients. HL7 is a basis for messaging that helps healthcare providers provide better care by ensuring interoperability. These international standards provide guidance for transferring and sharing data between various healthcare providers.

40

Nevertheless, health information is identified by a multiplicity of code values that may change based on the entity generating those results. This has downsides for the healthcare network that may need to implement various codes to access and manage information coming from multiple sources. For instance, managed care providers usually have negotiated contracts that reimburse episodes for care and unique coding to initiate automated claim payments. Associating each entity-specific code with its corresponding universal code can require a huge investment in both human and financial capital.

At the same time, a universal code system will help global facilities and departments receive and send results from their locations for comparison and consultation and may lead to a larger public health initiative of enhancing clinical outcomes and quality of care.

LOINC is one of the standards adopted in the U.S. federal government systems for the electronic exchange of clinical health information. In 1999, it was recognized by the HL7 standards development organization as the appropriate code set for laboratory test names in transactions between healthcare facilities, laboratories, laboratory testing devices, and public health authorities.

Content

LOINC terminology has two main parts:

- Laboratory LOINC: It includes laboratory tests, such as microbiology tests for antibiotic susceptibilities.

- Clinical LOINC: It includes several non-lab concepts (ECG concepts, cardiac echo, and obstetric ultrasound). Clinical LOINC has the following subparts:

  - Clinical documents: These are concepts for several types of clinical reports (e.g., discharge summary, well-child visit note).

  - Survey instruments: These are concepts for standardized surveys (e.g., Glasgow Coma Score, PHQ-9 depression scale).

Format

A formal, distinct, and unique six-part name is assigned to each term for the test or observation identity. The database presently has over 71,000 observation terms that can be obtained and understood universally. Each database record involves six fields for the unique specification of each identified single test, observation, or measurement:

- Component: What is measured, assessed, or observed (e.g., urea)

- Kind of property: Features of what is measured like length, mass, volume, time stamp, etc.

- Time aspect: The interval of time over which there was an observation or measurement

- System: The context or specimen type within which there was an observation (e.g., blood or urine)

- Type of scale: The scale of measure, which may be quantitative, ordinal, nominal, or narrative

- Type of method: The procedure used in making the measurement or observation

- A unique code: A unique code (format: nnnnn-n) is given to each entry upon registration. Other database fields involve status and mapping information for database change management, synonyms, related terms, and substance information. For example, the molar masses or CAS registry numbers are possible choices for indicating nominal scales or translations.

Uses

Some of the benefits from implementing LOINC may involve enhanced communication in integrated healthcare delivery networks, better community-wide electronic health records, the automatic transfer of case reports for reportable diseases to public health authorities for disease control or detection of epidemics, enhanced transfer of payment information for provided services, and a significant improvement in the entire quality of health care by minimizing errors in the system.

Since universal standards are being promoted (if not implemented) by national organizations and agencies, the dialogue will continue regarding

43

the development, structure, financing, monitoring, enforcement, and integration of standards within the broader healthcare system.

International interest in LOINC is growing. Several efforts have been undertaken to translate the LOINC documents and terms into different languages, including simplified Chinese, German, and Spanish. In January 2009, the software RELMA (Regenstrief LOINC Mapping Assistant) was accessible in separate downloads that have an additional word index in Spanish, simplified Chinese, or Korean, enabling searches in these languages as well as English. Harmonization efforts between LOINC and SNOMED CT started in 2012.

Key Takeaways

- The WHO manages the ICD as an international diagnostic tool for the classification of diseases.

- The ICD provides diagnostic codes for various health conditions, symptoms, and external causes of injury or disease.

- The most recent version, ICD-11, was released in January 2022 to achieve international compatability for health statistics.

- The ICD has a section for the classification of mental and behavioral disorders (Chapter V).

- Current Procedural Terminology (CPT) is a medical code set used to report medical procedures and services for billing purposes.

- CPT codes are categorized into evaluation and management (E/M), surgical, and radiology services.

- The HCPCS is a set of codes for billing and processing insurance claims.

- The HCPCS includes Level I (CPT) and Level II codes for non-physician services and supplies.

- SNOMED CT is a detailed clinical terminology system used to encode clinical concepts in health care.

- SNOMED CT can be used to improve communication among healthcare professionals for better patient care by providing a standardized language for clinical concepts.

If you want to acquire the required skills to be a pro medical biller and coder and earn more, read on in the next chapter.

CHAPTER 3: BUILDING ESSENTIAL SKILLS FOR MEDICAL BILLING AND CODING

Any field requires the proper skills for workers to function effectively, and medical billing and coding are no exception. In this chapter, you'll learn how to acquire analytical skills and attention to detail as well as engage in practical exercises, followed by developing familiarity with the technology and software with hands-on guidance. Then you'll develop an understanding of medical terminology with learning exercises and quizzes. Lastly, you will understand the ethical considerations and the importance of accuracy with relevant case studies and scenarios.

Analytical Skills and Attention to Detail: Practical Exercises

Medical coding and billing professionals need good analytical skills to analyze medical records and insurance claims, detect errors or discrepancies, and interpret insurance policies and procedures to ensure adherence to all regulations.

Attention to detail is also required since coders must accurately detect and interpret medical procedures and diagnoses. A small mistake in coding can escalate into huge errors in billing. This can result in lost revenue or even legal consequences, which is all the more reason they should be meticulous and precise during coding and billing exercises.

These practical exercises can boost the skills explained above:

- Case Studies: Analyze real-life scenarios by reviewing patient information, medical records, and encounter notes, as well as apply coding guidelines, select accurate codes, and ensure compliance with regulations.

- Coding Practice: Try exercises coding several medical encounters, like outpatient visits, surgeries, or diagnostic tests, as well as learning various code sets and effectively reading through coding manuals.

- Auditing and Documentation Reviews: Audit medical records and review documentation for completeness, accuracy, and support of billed services. Evaluate code assignment appropriateness and detect discrepancies or missing information.

- Reimbursement Analysis: Review claims and payment information to detect potential errors or discrepancies. Compare billed charges to reimbursement amounts to identify coding or billing issues that may affect reimbursement.

- Compliance and Regulatory Exercises: Learn and comply with coding guidelines and regulations. Focus on the correct use of modifiers, adherence to National Correct Coding Initiative (NCCI) edits, and guidelines set by regulatory bodies such as the CMS.

Regular practice of these exercises will enhance accuracy, efficiency, and adherence to regulations in medical billing and coding. Get feedback from experts and engage in coding workshops for more skill enhancement and detection of areas for improvement.

Familiarity with Technology and Software: Hands-On Guidance

Familiarity with technology and software is an essential skill for medical billing and coding professionals. The healthcare industry depends on digital systems and electronic health records (EHRs), so it is essential to have hands-on experience and proficiency with different software applications. Below are some key points to try when building comfort with technology and software:

- Get Used to EHR Systems: Understand and become a pro with the EHR software used in your organization by learning how to navigate the system, input and retrieve data, and use important features.

- Try Coding Software: Get used to coding software applications like encoders or coding-specific modules within EHR systems. Practice using these tools to boost efficiency and accuracy in coding tasks.

- Be Current on Industry Tools and Technology: Strive to learn about the latest tools and advancements in medical billing and coding. Attend industry events and consider training opportunities to understand emerging software applications.

- Seek Training and Hands-On Guidance: Receive training and guidance from experienced professionals or your organization's IT department if you are a newbie to specific software. Optimize any training provided by your employer or consider online courses.

- Practice and Experiment: Explore various features and functionalities of software applications. Be proactive in seeking opportunities to apply your technical skills.

By developing familiarity and comfort with technology and software, you will improve your efficiency and accuracy in medical billing and coding. Consider the digital transformation in health care and keep increasing your knowledge and proficiency in needed applications.

Understanding of Medical Terminology: Learning Exercises and Quizzes

Understanding Medical Terminology

There are several relevant terms you'll want to get used to as you learn more about coding. Below are some of them:

- CATEGORY (CPT): The CPT code set is sectioned into three categories. Category I, which is the biggest and most commonly used, explains medical procedures, technologies, and services. Category II is applied for performance management and additional data. Category III contains the codes for new and experimental medical procedures and services.

- CATEGORY (ICD): In ICD, the category is the first three characters of the code, and it describes the basic manifestation of the injury or sickness. In some cases, only this category can be used to describe the condition of the patient accurately. Nevertheless, the coder must regularly list a more detailed description of the injury or illness (see subcategory and subclassification). Note that categories are three numbers in ICD-10-CM.

- CLINICAL MODIFICATION: The clinical modification (CM) designation, developed by the National Center for Health Statistics, is added to the ICD code sets upon their implementation in the United States. Many countries improve and clarify ICD code sets when they use them. For example, the US expanded the ICD-10 from 14,000 codes to over 68,000 individual codes. This term is abbreviated "-CM" and is added at the end of the ICD code title. For example, you can read the ICD-10-CM as "International Classification of Diseases, Tenth Revision, Clinical Modification."

- CMS: CMS is the Center for Medicare and Medicaid Services. This federal agency updates and manages the HCPCS code set and is currently one of the most relevant organizations in health care.

- CPT: CPT is the current procedural terminology. Released, copyrighted, and managed by the American Medical Association, CPT is a huge set of codes that explains the procedure or service carried out on a patient. This code is divided into three categories, of which the first category is the most relevant and common. CPT codes are an important part of the reimbursement process. These codes are five characters long and may be numeric or alphanumeric.

- HCPCS: Healthcare Common Procedure Coding System, pronounced "hick-picks," is the major procedural code set for reporting procedures to Medicare, Medicaid, and several other third-party payers. Managed by the CMS, HCPCS is divided into two levels. Level I is similar to CPT and is used similarly. Level II explains the equipment, medication, and outpatient services not involved in CPT.

- E-CODES: E-codes are a collection of ICD-10-CM codes that involve codes for external causes of injury, such as auto accidents, poisoning, and homicide.

- EVALUATION AND MANAGEMENT (CPT): Evaluation and Management, or E&M, is a section of CPT codes for explaining the assessment of a patient's health and the management of their care. For example, the codes for visits to the doctor's office and trips to the emergency room are added to E&M. You will find

51

E&M at the front of the CPT manual, irrespective of being out of numerical order. The codes for E&M are 99201–99499.

- ICD: The International Classification of Diseases is a collection of medical diagnostic codes founded over a century ago. Managed today by the WHO, ICD codes offer a universal language for reporting diseases and injuries. Presently, we use ICD-10-CM. ICD codes are numeric or alphanumeric. They include a three-character category, which explains the injury or disease and which is usually followed by a decimal point and two-to-four more characters based on the code set. These characters provide more details about the manifestation and location of the disease.

- MODIFIER: A modifier is a two-character code that is included in a procedure code to show a relevant variation that does not, by itself, change the definition of the procedure. CPT codes have numeric modifiers, whereas HCPCS codes have alphanumeric modifiers. These are included at the end of a code and are preceded by a hyphen and may offer details about the procedure itself, that procedure's Medicare eligibility, and many other relevant facets. For instance, the CPT modifier -51 alerts the payer that this procedure was one of multiple procedures. However, the HCPCS modifier -LT describes a bilateral procedure that was carried out only on the left side of the body.

- MODIFIER EXEMPT (CPT): Specific codes in CPT cannot have modifiers included in them. This is just a short list and is located in the appendices of the CPT manual.

- NCHS: The National Center for Health Statistics is a government agency that monitors health information and creates and releases both the clinical modifications to ICD codes and their annual updates.

- PATHOLOGY: Pathology is the science of the causes and effects of disease.

- SUBCATEGORY: In ICD codes, the subcategory explains the digit that follows the decimal point. This digit further explains the nature of the illness or injury and provides more details regarding its location or manifestation.

- SUBCLASSIFICATION: The subclassification comes after the subcategory in ICD codes. The subclassification further expands on the subcategory and provides more details concerning the manifestation, severity, or location of the injury or disease. ICD-10-CM also has a subclassification that explains which encounter this is for the doctor, whether this is a first treatment for the sickness, a follow-up, or the evaluation of a condition resulting from a past injury or disease. You may find as many as three subclassification characters in ICD-10-CM.

- TECHNICAL COMPONENT: This is part of a medical procedure that focuses on only the technical aspect of the procedure, not the interpretative or professional aspect. A technical component might involve the administration of a chest X-ray, yet it would not add the evaluation of that X-ray for disease or abnormality.

- WHO: The World Health Organization is an international body and an agency of the United Nations that oversees the development of ICD codes and is one of the most relevant organizations in international health.

- Z-CODES: These codes explain situations outside of injury or disease that make a patient visit a health professional. For example, this might include a patient visiting a doctor because of their family medical history.

Learning Exercises and Quizzes

Below are some learning exercises and quizzes that help to build proficiency in medical terminology:

- Flashcards: Create flashcards with medical terms on one side and their definitions or meanings on the opposite side. Consistently review the flashcards to strengthen your knowledge and enhance recall. Moreover, you can create sets of flashcards based on certain medical specialties or body systems to emphasize specific terminology.

- Word Association: Try to associate medical terms with their corresponding meanings or related terms. This exercise helps create connections between different medical terms for better understanding and retention. For instance, associate "cardiology" with "heart" and "dermatology" with "skin."

- Prefixes, Suffixes, and Root Words: Study common prefixes, suffixes, and root words used in medical terminology. Learning the meanings of these word parts enables you to interpret the whole meaning of a medical term. Try to break down medical terms into their components to understand their individual meanings.

- Medical Terminology Quizzes: Try online quizzes or use medical terminology textbooks with quizzes to test your knowledge and understanding. These quizzes include multiple-choice, fill-in-the-blank, or matching exercises and questions. They offer an interactive way to evaluate your progress and detect areas you should improve.

- Case Studies and Documentation Analysis: Try reading case studies or analyzing medical documentation to identify and interpret medical terms. Read medical reports, like laboratory results, physician notes, and radiology reports, to get more of an idea of real-world terminology usage, and your knowledge of medical terms will increase within the context of patient care.

- Medical Terminology Resources: Use resources such as medical dictionaries, textbooks, and online databases to understand medical terminology, as well as learn commonly used terms in different medical specialties.

Don't forget to keep practicing and reviewing medical terminology to strengthen your understanding and enhance your proficiency. Building a strong foundation in medical terminology will significantly improve your ability to accurately assign codes and communicate effectively in the field of medical billing and coding.

Ethical Considerations and the Importance of Accuracy: Case Studies and Scenarios

Ethical Considerations and the Importance of Accuracy

Working in medical billing and coding includes learning about the standards of professionalism and ethical behavior required in this type of healthcare job. Medical billing and coding specialists can access confidential and highly sensitive patient information, which makes a dedication to professionalism paramount. Below are some of the standards medical billers and coders should comply with every time:

- Data Gathering

The manner of gathering data through coding practices can develop into an ethical issue. Medical billing and coding specialists should accurately and consistently gather data. All data required for coding should be reported for accuracy. These healthcare workers should comply with all internal coding policies and procedures on data gathering and reporting and prevent changing or concealing any coded information.

- Accuracy

Medical coders should always be accurate when coding and prevent inputting codes for medical services, procedures, diagnoses, or treatments that haven't been used or done. Maintaining top-notch accuracy is one of the most relevant standards of professionalism for medical billers and coders. Not complying with this standard can expose these healthcare workers to accusations of fraud and potentially affect patient safety, for instance, if the wrong treatment or diagnosis is coded.

- Misrepresenting or Changing Data

Medical billers and coders should always avoid changing or misrepresenting data when coding a patient's procedure, diagnosis, service, or treatment. If a patient or physician requests changes to be made that do not fit the clinical documentation—for instance, when a patient wants to ensure their insurance will cover a procedure—medical billers and coders should not comply. This involves deliberately entering incorrect codes or including codes that are not part of the patient's documentation.

- Overbilling

Overbilling can result in higher medical bills for patients and make insurance companies deny reimbursement. Medical billing and coding specialists should not bill for services, treatments, or procedures that aren't deemed billable. When in doubt, check the details of the patient's care with the physician(s) for accurate billing and coding. For instance, every portion of a procedure might not be deemed billable unless the physician states otherwise. Clarifying these challenging scenarios with physicians helps minimize the risk of overbilling.

- Bad Coding

Medical billing and coding specialists should work hard to prevent making errors that lead to bad coding. For instance, specialists should prevent upcoding or undercoding, which involves coding for a more costly service than what was offered or for a less costly service when a more costly one was performed. Moreover, medical billing and coding specialists should also prevent unbundling, which means using separate codes instead of one code for a whole group of procedures or treatments.

- Maintaining Professional Values

Medical billing and coding specialists should maintain professional values and motivate colleagues to follow that path as well. This might include revealing unethical behavior that a colleague has engaged in or discouraging colleagues from misbehaving. Furthermore, medical coders and billers should understand the standards of professionalism assigned to them. They should also learn the correct procedures and policies for reporting unethical behavior.

- Patient Confidentiality

HIPAA legally requires healthcare workers and providers to manage patient confidentiality. Moreover, safeguarding patients' information is an ethical issue. Medical billing and coding specialists can come across sensitive information on patients' records, which should always be kept confidential. These workers should also avoid accessing any medical information that isn't relevant to the treatment, service, or procedure they're handling in medical billing and coding.

- Honesty and Integrity

Honesty and integrity are important parts of medical professionalism. Medical billing and coding professionals should always act with integrity and honesty. This means refusing to engage in unethical practices or behaviors in coding, such as misrepresenting data or breaching patient confidentiality by looking up irrelevant patient information. Therefore, integrity and honesty should be prioritized when making ethical choices on the job and maintaining high standards of professionalism, even when pressured to act otherwise.

Case Studies and Scenarios

Case studies provide real-world situations for medical billing and coding professionals to tackle ethical issues. By analyzing these cases, professionals better understand ethical implications and their solutions. Case studies also involve accuracy in medical billing and coding, as inaccuracies can result in financial loss and compromised patient care.

Scenarios offer hypothetical situations to practice decision-making skills, emphasizing ethical considerations and expecting professionals to assess conflicting priorities and maintain patient confidentiality. Practicing case studies and scenarios enables critical thinking, problem-solving abilities, and ethical decision-making to help professionals detect potential ethical challenges and make informed decisions that conform to legal requirements and professional standards.

This scenario includes a patient presenting for a follow-up visit with symptoms of type 2 diabetes. See if you can select the correct codes.

Clinical Scenario

Chief Complaint

- The patient, a 52-year-old male, visited the office for follow-up of type 2 diabetes mellitus (T2DM), hyperlipidemia, hypertension, and urine microalbumin. The patient reports he was diagnosed with T2DM at age 45. The patient has been on insulin since 2010. Hence, after the last visit, the patient reports blood sugars are stable.

Current Treatment:

- Current diabetic regimen involves Tresiba 36 units daily and Xigduo (5/1000mg) 2 tablets daily.

- Reviewed medication list—medication compliance is okay.

- Glucose records reviewed

- Blood glucose monitoring is carried out 0–1 time daily.

- The patient disclaims hypoglycemia or hypoglycemia symptoms (i.e., no dizziness, sweating, confusion, or headaches).

Diet/Exercise/Weight:

- Patient is overweight but usually consumes a healthy diet and visits the gym two to three times per week.

Diabetic Related Complications:

- Neuropathy symptoms: Positive stocking/glove numbness or tingling. No mononeuropathy and postprandial bloating

- Retinopathy: Up-to-date on routine surveillance. First diagnosed 1/22/2018

- Nephropathy: Positive. Up-to-date on routine surveillance

Review of Systems

- Constitutional/Endocrine/Musculoskeletal: Negative

Social History

- Smoking status: Does not smoke

Physical Exam

- BP: 140/82

- Pulse: 78

- Weight: 271 lb 12.8 oz (123.3 kg)

- BMI: Body mass index is 36.86 kg/m²

- General: Alert; NAD with normal affect

- Eyes: EOMI; no icterus

- HENT: Atraumatic; oropharynx clear with moist mucous membranes

- Neck: Supple, normal size thyroid, no palpable nodules

- Respiratory: Normal respiratory effort

- Cardiovascular: Regular rate and rhythm; no edema

- Musculoskeletal: FROM; no synovitis

- Neurological: Reflexes 2+ at biceps, relaxation phase normal; no tremor

- Skin: No rash; no ulcerations

- Diabetic Foot Exam: No lesions; good pulses

Assessment

Type 2 diabetes mellitus with hyperglycemia with long-term ongoing use of insulin

- Type 2 diabetes mellitus with polyneuropathy

- Type 2 diabetes mellitus with microalbuminuria, with long-term ongoing use of insulin

- Type 2 diabetes, uncontrolled, with retinopathy

- Class 2 severe obesity due to excess calories with severe comorbidity and BMI of 36.0 to 36.9 in adult

- Hyperlipidemia related to type 2 diabetes mellitus

- Hypertension related to diabetes

- Vitamin D deficiency

Documentation Coding Requirements

When documenting diabetes, add the following:

- Type:

  - Type 1

63

- Type 2

    - Due to underlying condition

    - Drug or chemical induced diabetes mellitus

    - Diabetes mellitus in pregnancy, childbirth, and the puerperium

- With or without complication

- With or without coma

    - Eye:

        - Left Right Bilateral

        - Diagnosis Codes

        - E11.65 Type 2 diabetes mellitus with hyperglycemia

        - E11.42 Type 2 diabetes mellitus with diabetic polyneuropathy

        - E11.29 Type 2 diabetes mellitus with other diabetic kidney complication

        - E11.319 Type 2 diabetes with unspecified diabetic retinopathy with macular edema

64

- E11.69 Type 2 diabetes mellitus with other specified complication

- E11.59 Type 2 diabetes mellitus with other circulatory complications

- E66.01 Morbid (severe) obesity due to excess calories

- Z68.36 BMI 36.0-36.9, adult

- Z79.4 Long term (current) use of insulin

- E55.9 Vitamin D deficiency, unspecified

- R80.9 Proteinuria, unspecified

- E78.5 Hyperlipidemia, unspecified

Key Takeaways

- Medical billing and coding professionals should acquire analytical skills and attention to detail.

- Practical exercises like case studies, coding practice, auditing, and reimbursement analysis can improve your analytical skills and attention to detail.

- Familiarity with technology and software will benefit medical billers and coders, and hands-on guidance will improve proficiency.

- You should learn medical terminology and practice exercises and quizzes to improve proficiency.

- Consider ethical considerations and accuracy in medical billing and coding, as well as case studies and scenarios, to understand the importance of professionalism and ethical behavior.

- Data gathering, accuracy, avoiding misrepresentation or changing data, avoiding overbilling, and maintaining patient confidentiality are relevant ethical considerations.

- Professionals should also be honest, have integrity, and comply with professional values in their work.

For many reasons, you need to be certified as a medical biller and coder, and the next chapter will enlighten you about the reasons and benefits of obtaining certifications. Keep reading to learn more.

CHAPTER 4: GETTING EDUCATED AND CERTIFIED

An individual working on getting their certification in coding and billing shows they are the professional a medical company would benefit from having on their team. The medical field needs individuals with knowledge on billing and coding and understanding the insurance world, ensuring proper reimbursement on claims.

—Diana Murphy, Instructor, Penn Foster's Medical Billing and Coding Program

In this chapter, we will explore the educational requirements needed and options available as a medical biller and coder. Then, we'll progress to understanding the importance and process of certification and finally to comparing different certification bodies and their exams. Let's get started.

Overview of Educational Requirements and Options

There are many education options available to people pursuing training in this field. Some medical billers and coders hold a two-year associate's degree or a bachelor's degree; however, this is not always required. Several schools provide medical and billing coding paths, such as diplomas, certificates, and degree programs.

Certificate and Diploma Programs

Certificate and diploma programs usually require between nine months to one year to complete. Career colleges, community colleges, professional organizations, and stand-alone services provide these programs. However, career college programs generally have a quicker time for completion.

- Prerequisites: High school diploma or GED, minimum scores on standardized tests like ACT or SAT

- Courses/curriculum: Anatomy and physiology, medical terminology, patient privacy, disease classification, and coding

- Considerations: Take note of the coding system(s) the program teaches because some are focused on hospital coding or physician's office coding systems.

- Time to complete: 9–12 months

Associate's Degree Programs

An associate's degree requires more time than a medical billing and coding certificate or diploma since the curriculum exceeds just the essential information for billing and coding careers. Both career colleges and community colleges provide associate's degree programs.

- Prerequisites: High school diploma or GED, minimum GPA (often 2.0 or above). Some programs expect prerequisite coursework like anatomy and physiology.

- Courses/curriculum: Medical terminology, pharmacology, diagnostic coding, procedural coding, and ethics

- Considerations: If you wish to get more education, including a bachelor's or master's degree, you can transfer credits from your associate's degree.

- Time to complete: Two years

Bachelor's Degree Programs

Earning a bachelor's degree before becoming a medical biller and coder means that you'll probably major in health information management or healthcare administration. Apart from the classes in your major, you should complete general education requirements.

Based on whether you earn a Bachelor of Science or Bachelor of Arts, you'll complete coursework in general sciences or liberal arts. A bachelor's degree can apply to a broad range of career options within the healthcare field.

- Prerequisites: High school diploma or GED and minimum scores on standardized examinations like ACT or SAT. The application process may also involve essay questions, recommendations, and interviews with admissions staff.

- Courses/curriculum: Health information management, healthcare delivery systems, medical terminology, healthcare reimbursement, personnel management, anatomy, and physiology

- Considerations: If you desire to pursue management positions later, a bachelor's degree will come in handy. Several bachelor's degrees in this field expect in-field work experience like internships.

- Time to complete: Four years

Online Courses

Online options for diploma, certificate, associate's degree, and bachelor's degree programs are growing in popularity. This is an advantage for anyone who can't fit traditional, in-person programs into their lives.

Online and in-person programs cover identical content. They will both teach you the medical basics required—medical terminology, for example—and train you in a coding system or systems.

- Where they differ: Online programs are known for their flexibility, making them popular among students who are working simultaneously, offering caregiver support, or managing other responsibilities. As you explore your education options, you'll want to decide if online medical billing and coding programs are perfect for you.

Certification

After earning a degree or completing a medical billing and coding program, you can decide to earn a certification. Certifications can be general or specific, based on what competencies you want to show. For instance, you can earn certification in foundational coding, or you can delve deeper into a narrower topic like anesthesia or obstetrics and gynecology so that employers can see that you've not only studied a niche topic but have shown your expertise.

Salary

Just like most fields, pay for medical billers and coders differs based on your experience, educational level, certifications, location, and medical setting where you work. Therefore, medical billers and coders are professionals who are compensated based on those factors. As you ponder what type of education to pursue, consider your salary expectations and explore strategies to increase your pay.

The Importance and Process of Certification

Importance of Certification

While you can pursue careers in medical billing and coding without professional certifications, certification indicates that a person has been properly trained with the knowledge and skills required to be a proficient medical coder or biller. Below are some top reasons to get certified:

- Higher earnings: The AAPC salary reports show that Certified Professional Coders (CPC) earn 20% more than their noncertified counterparts.

- Greater employability: Although the medical coding and billing field is expanding at an above-average rate with 15% projected growth by 2024, it is a competitive market. Most employers seek professionals with at least one certification or who can get certified shortly after hire.

- Opportunities for advancement: Becoming certified, particularly in several coding specialties, enables professionals to progress into new job positions more easily and shows employers a commitment to continuing education and the entire field. This commitment is rewarding. In 2015, AAPC members with two or more certifications earned 24.5% more than those with only one. Meanwhile, members with three or more certifications earned nearly 40% more than those with only one.

- Professional connections: Although becoming a member of certification-granting organizations is not often compulsory to become certified, membership does create connections to other medical coding and billing professionals. Connecting with

72

individuals and groups who know and respect professional certifications and education can result in several opportunities.

- Personal growth: The benefits attached to passing a certification exam go beyond just those for potential employers. Certified individuals can trust the accuracy of their work, and training for certifications results in new knowledge and growth as a professional.

Process of Certification

Getting any kind of industry certification requires you to prove your knowledge by passing an exam given by a major certifying body (eligibility requirements may apply). The AAPC administers the Certified Professional Coder (CPC®) exam, which contains three of the healthcare industry's most frequently used code sets.

To attain full CPC status, candidates must pass the exam. The next step is to get either two years of work experience or 80 contact hours of a coding preparation course in addition to one year of on-the-job experience. Individuals who pass the exam but don't yet meet the full eligibility requirements will receive the CPC Apprentice (CPC-A) designation, which can be upgraded to full CPC status when they provide proof of experience.

1. The CPC Examination

The CPC certification exam includes 100 multiple-choice questions. It helps to assess the candidate's knowledge of anatomy, medical terminology, laboratory and clinical procedures, practice management, coding guidelines, etc. It also assesses how well the candidate can apply the proper procedure, supply, and diagnosis codes.

Individuals who sit for the exam can use approved manuals for reference and may require up to four hours to complete it.

2. Getting Certified

Whether you desire to be a coder, a biller, or in a hybrid role that manages both tasks, earning your CPC or CPC-A credential demonstrates your proficiency in comprehending medical terminology and the industry's universal coding systems.

Note that this is a process that will require some work, so be prepared to participate in the long game. Don't forget that you want to advance your career, so be committed to doing it right.

3. Complete Your Education

The initial step to a medical coding and billing career can begin with getting your education.

If you are aware of the kind of healthcare setting you want to work in, consider reviewing local job postings to see what employers desire when hiring medical coders and billers.

Do they want candidates with a certificate or a diploma? Do they value individuals with an associate's degree? Is certification needed or strongly preferred? This will give you a hint about where to begin.

4. Choose a Diploma or Degree Program

Several employers don't require a degree for entry-level medical coding and billing jobs, yet some may prefer candidates with some kind of formal training in medical terminology, standard industry codes, and essential software. Obtaining credentials from an accredited health education school demonstrates preparation for this field.

A diploma program mainly focuses on important healthcare classes like coding, computers, records management, claims processing, and medical terminology—and generally can be completed in less than a year based on the speed of the individual student.

An associate's degree is usually a two-year program; however, at some schools, it will only require about a year and a half, depending on the speed of the individual student and the program itself.

The degree curriculum probably includes the same classes as the diploma program, with additional courses like English, math, sociology, biology, etc., to help enhance and broaden students' skills.

Furthermore, you may also select from campus-based courses or online learning. Although students preparing for clinical roles, like nursing assistants or phlebotomy technicians, are required to take on-campus

75

courses, computer-based work such as coding and billing is perfect for an online learning environment.

Lastly, if you want to pursue medical coding and billing certification before applying for jobs, you should choose a diploma or degree program that will prepare you for industry certification like the CPC designation. Even if you temporarily lack the work experience to attain full CPC status, you can still add the CPC-A designation to your résumé after passing the exam.

5. Approved Exam Materials

Candidates could not possibly memorize the many thousands of codes used in this field, so the AAPC allows applicants to reference approved manuals during the exam. Note that only hard-copy manuals are allowed, as electronic devices are prohibited in the exam room.

For the Certified Professional Coder exam, you can bring the following approved manuals with you:

- Current Procedural Terminology: CPT books (AMA standard or professional edition only)

- International Classification of Diseases: Your choice of ICD-10-CM code book

- Healthcare Common Procedure Coding System: Your choice of HCPCS Level II code book

6. What Does the Certification Exam Cover?

The CPC exam is open book. You will be given four hours to complete 100 multiple-choice questions. You will need a score of 70% or higher to pass. The categories tested are the following:

- Integumentary Surgical Coding

- Respiratory Surgical Coding

- Nervous System Surgical Coding

- Endocrine System Surgical Coding

- Digestive System Surgical Coding

- Urinary System Surgical Coding

- Musculoskeletal System Surgical Coding

- Mediastinum & Diaphragm Surgical Coding

- Male/Female Genital Surgical Coding

- Hemic & Lymphatic Surgical Coding

- Maternity & Delivery

- Eye & Ocular Adnexa Surgical Coding

- ICD-10-CM

- HCPCS Level II

- Radiology

- Pathology

- Laboratory

- Medicine

- Anesthesia

- Evaluation and Management

- Anatomy and Physiology

- Medical Terminology

- Coding Guidelines

- Practice Management

After completing the CPC exam, you'll get the results within seven to ten business days. You can check out the results online in your "My AAPC" account, and you'll get the hard copy via email. The exam fee includes one free retake (if required). After earning a passing score, you can add the CPC-A certification to your résumé.

Comparison of Different Certification Bodies and Their Exams

No specific certification is deemed the "best" overall. Each type of billing and coding certification has its pros and cons and different requirements. It's more about selecting which certification best suits your goals and knowing which certifications you can take. Although there are several coding-specific certifications—even certifications for coding specialties—the most common exams include:

1. Certified Billing and Coding Specialist (CBCS) Exam

The Certified Billing and Coding Specialist (CBCS) certification provided by the National Healthcareer Association (NHA) helps to ensure that medical billing and coding professionals learn the right way to code for illnesses, procedures, and other common medical needs that complies with insurance standards. The CBCS includes broad, foundational skills that are relevant to medical billers and coders who desire to work in physician's offices, hospitals, dental offices, nursing homes, insurance companies, and other medical facilities.

The exam requires about three hours to complete and has 100 scored questions; there is a time limit. Register on the NHA website if you want to take the exam. Then you can take the test at a testing center close by or remotely. Some programs, such as the Penn Foster Medical Billing and Coding Program, include the cost of the exam in their students' tuition. In addition, prep materials are added for better preparation to pass the test and get certified.

- CBCS requirements: Sitting for the CBCS requires you to be at least 18 years old and to have a high school diploma or its equivalent. Also, you must have completed a medical billing and coding training program within the last five years or have at least one year of supervised work experience in the field.

- Who is the CBCS right for? The CBCS exam is a useful certification for anyone new to the medical billing and coding field with the desire to validate a wide range of relevant, foundational coding skills.

2. Certified Professional Coder (CPC) Exam

The Certified Professional Coder (CPC) certification provided by the AAPC is the most common medical billing and coding certification pursued by students. The CPC focuses on outpatient coding and covers how to assign diagnoses, procedures, and medical codes for several clinical services and cases.

The exam has 100 multiple-choice questions, and test takers have up to four hours to complete the exam. You can register to take the exam at a testing center nearby or online. For the online option, a reliable internet connection and an external webcam are required. The AAPC provides a free exam retake, and many students participate in their local AAPC chapters.

- CPC requirements: Sitting for the CPC exam requires you to be at least 18 years old and have a high school diploma. Moreover,

80

you should have an active membership with AAPC; individuals taking the exam must have relevant work experience or education before taking the test.

- Who is the CPC right for? The CPC exam is beneficial for people who want to be a member of the AAPC, which provides networking opportunities and webinars to further their education.

3. Certified Coding Associate (CCA) Exam

The CCA certification provided by the American Health Information Management Association (AHIMA) contains every coding across different settings, such as hospitals and physicians' offices. This medical coding and billing certification verifies your skills in coding procedures for recordkeeping, compliance, and confidentiality. The CCA exam has a time limit of two hours and has 105 total questions.

- CCA requirements: There is no minimum age requirement to be eligible to take the CCA certification exam. Sitting for the exam requires you to have a high school diploma or equivalent. AHIMA expects you also to have either six months of experience in the field or to have completed an approved training course before taking the test, but it's not compulsory.

- Who is the CCA right for? The CCA exam is perfect for entry-level medical billers and coders who have not completed an approved training course or those who are novices in the field.

Is the CBCS a Good Certification?

Yes, it is a good certification for a medical biller and coder to have. Earning the CBCS credential shows that you have the needed foundational skills in coding and health care and that you will be valuable to any healthcare organization.

The Differences between the CPC, the CBCS, and the CCA

Note: Employers don't usually prefer one medical billing and coding certification over another, so you should select one certification (at least at first) that best suits you. Learning the similarities and differences between the exams can help you choose wisely.

The CPC and CCA are multipurpose certifications that can be used across multiple settings, while the CBCS may be more appealing to employers in the insurance industry. All three exams demand a high school diploma or equivalent, with the CPC and CBCS recommending a minimum age of 18. They are all great starting points for students who decide they want to pursue a career in inpatient coding.

Other differences are exam cost and experience requirements.

Key Takeaways

- Several educational options are available for individuals pursuing a career in medical billing and coding, such as certificate, diploma, associate's degree, and bachelor's degree programs.

- Certificate and diploma programs can be completed within 9–12 months and include courses like anatomy and physiology, medical terminology, disease classification, and coding.

- Associate degree programs provide more detailed education and usually require two years to complete. Their courses include medical terminology, pharmacology, diagnostic coding, procedural coding, and ethics.

- Bachelor's degree programs, like the ones in health information management or healthcare administration, offer a broader education and can result in different career options within the healthcare field. They typically require four years to complete.

- Online courses are growing very common and provide flexibility for individuals who cannot attend in-person programs.

- Certification is not compulsory; however, it can be useful in terms of higher earnings, greater employability, opportunities for advancement, professional connections, and personal growth.

- The certification process generally includes passing an exam administered by a certifying body. The CPC exam, provided by the AAPC, is among the most common exams in the field.

- Various certification bodies provide exams with their own requirements and specialties, like the CBCS exam offered by the NHA and the CCA exam offered by the AHIMA.

- The selection of the certification to pursue is based on individual goals and choice. Each certification has its pros and cons, and you should select one that best matches your career objectives.

- Salary in the medical billing and coding field differs based on experience, education, certifications, location, and work setting. Considering salary expectations and exploring strategies to boost pay are relevant when deciding on education and certification options.

If you want to explore practical medical coding exercises and examples, then let's move on to the next chapter.

CHAPTER 5: PRACTICAL CODING: EXERCISES AND EXAMPLES

Welcome to this chapter. Sit back and relax as we take you through hands-on exercises for coding common medical scenarios, a step-by-step breakdown of coding complex medical cases, and detailed examples of coding using different coding systems.

Hands-On Exercises for Coding Common Medical Scenarios

Quality clinical documentation leads to effective communication, medical necessity confirmation, and accurate code selection. Below are outpatient scenarios coded in ICD-10-CM and ICD-9-CM to discuss documentation and coding nuances in your specialty. Note that these scenarios are illustrative, so don't take them as strict guidelines due to variations in patient history and circumstances. Nevertheless, only a subset of relevant codes is indicated to emphasize specific topics.

FAMILY PRACTICE CLINICAL SCENARIOS:

Scenario 1: Abdominal Pain

SCENARIO DETAILS

CHIEF COMPLAINT

- "My stomach aches, and I feel full of gas."

HISTORY

- A 47-year-old male with mid-abdominal epigastric pain is experiencing severe nausea and vomiting. He can't retain any food or liquid. The pain is now "severe" and regular.

- In the last month, he has had an estimated 13-pound weight loss.

- The patient said he ate 12 sausages at the Sunday church breakfast five days ago, which he feels is the cause of his predicament.

- The patient also said he has been using alcohol. He consumes five–six beers daily now, down from 10–12 daily six months ago, which made him have nausea and sweats with "the shakes" when he did not drink.

EXAM

- VS: T 99.8°F, otherwise normal

- Mild jaundice noted

- The upper abdomen is swollen and sensitive to touch, with a noticeable stiffness. You can also notice protective muscle tension, and bowel sounds are faint in every aspect of the abdomen.

- Oral mucosa dry, chapped lips, decreased skin turgor

ASSESSMENT AND PLAN

- Dehydration and suspected acute pancreatitis

- The patient was admitted to the hospital. The relevant orders were promptly documented and relayed to the on-call hospitalists.

- 1L IV NS started in the office, and blood was taken for labs.

- Provided behavioral health counseling for substance abuse assessment and potential treatment.

- The patient's wife was updated about the plan, and she will go to the hospital by private vehicle.

SUMMARY OF ICD-10-CM IMPACTS

CLINICAL DOCUMENTATION

- Discuss the pain without ambiguity based on location.

- Alcohol-related disorders should be distinguished between alcohol use, alcohol abuse, and alcohol dependence. ICD-10-CM has changed the terminology and the criteria for coding substance abuse disorders. In this encounter note, as acute pancreatitis is suspected and the patient's alcohol intake status is documented, the corresponding alcoholism code is included.

- Abdominal tenderness can be assigned a unique code for documentation purposes. Normally, the documentation should show the presence of tenderness in the right or left upper quadrant, as well as the presence or absence of rebound tenderness, to foster the assignment of a more specific code. Presently, the ICD-10 code would be R10.819, abdominal tenderness unspecified site, as the documentation does not have much laterality and specificity.

CODING

ICD-9-CM DIAGNOSIS CODES

- 789.06 Abdominal pain, epigastric

- 789.60 Abdominal tenderness, unspecified site

- 782.4 Jaundice NOS

- 276.51 Dehydration

- 303.90 Other and unspecified alcohol dependence, unspecified drinking behavior

ICD-10-CM DIAGNOSIS CODES

- R10.13 Epigastric pain

- R10.819 Abdominal tenderness, unspecified site

- R17 Unspecified jaundice

- E86.0 Dehydration

- F10.20 Alcohol dependence, uncomplicated

OTHER IMPACTS

- No specific impacts were noted.

Scenario 2: Annual Physical Exam

SCENARIO DETAILS

CHIEF COMPLAINT

- "I'm here for my yearly check-up."

HISTORY

- The patient is a 73-year-old male who has been suffering from coronary artery disease, stent placement, hyperlipidemia, HTN, and GERD.

- He has been admitted to a hospital after a hypertensive crisis and discharged home on olmesartan medoxomil 20 mg daily.

- The patient stopped taking olmesartan medoxomil due to adverse side effects as well as persistent headache and fatigue he suffered after taking the medication.

- He usually walks, plays golf, and has an active social life. He doesn't complain of chest pain or dyspnea on exertion.

- The last colonoscopy was done nine months ago. However, there was no relevant pathology apart from having diverticular disease.

- Medications were reviewed.

EXAM

- His chest is clear, heart sounds normal, and his mental status exam is stable.

- The EKG indicates no changes compared to the previous one.

- Vital signs: The patient's blood pressure is 159/95 (elevated), but other vital signs are within normal limits. The patient noted that he could control his blood pressure with medication, but it increased after stopping the medication.

- BUN/creatinine normal limits.

ASSESSMENT AND PLAN

- Hypertension (HTN) was observed during today's examination, so we will switch from olmesartan medoxomil to metoprolol tartrate at a daily dose of 50 mg. The dosage will be adjusted every two weeks until the patient's blood pressure normalizes.

- He said he understood the instructions concerning daily home BP monitoring, consuming a low-sodium diet, and taking BP medication.

- We will follow up in two weeks to evaluate how effective the new BP medication therapy is and repeat the BUN/creatinine test.

SUMMARY OF ICD-10-CM IMPACTS

CLINICAL DOCUMENTATION

- Document the cause of the encounter: for administrative purposes, the assigned code may differ depending on the type of visit, such as screening without any reported complaints or suspected diagnoses. In such a scenario, give the patient an encounter without any reported complaints or suspected diagnoses.

- Document that the patient is not following the prescribed medication. Also, code for "underdosing" in such a scenario and document why the patient stopped taking the medications as well as whether a medical condition that is relevant to the encounter is the cause of the underdosing, and make sure there is a connection. Note that the ICD-10-CM codes provide more detailed information compared to the ICD-9-CM code V15.81, which shows a history of previous noncompliance. In this case, there was no documented history of noncompliance, and the side effects of taking the medication are headaches, which is still a patient complaint for this encounter. When documenting headaches, ensure to differentiate if they are intractable versus not intractable.

CODING

ICD-9-CM DIAGNOSIS CODES

- V70.0 Routine medical exam

- 401.9 Unspecified essential hypertension

- 339.3 Drug-induced headache, not elsewhere classified

ICD-10-CM DIAGNOSIS CODES

- Z00.01 Encounter for general adult medical examination with abnormal findings

- I10 Essential (primary) hypertension

- G44.40 Drug-induced headache, not elsewhere classified, not intractable

- T46.5X6A Underdosing of other antihypertensive drugs, initial encounter

- Z91.128 Patient's intentional underdosing of medication regimen for other reason

OTHER IMPACTS

- Check if the new patient-centric preventative health incentives for yearly exams are related to your practice.

- Within Medicare Advantage risk adjustment plans, you can use specific diagnosis codes to evaluate the severity of illness, risk factors, and resource utilization, operating under the framework of the hierarchical condition categories (HCC). Note that the impacts of HCC are usually not accounted for during the conversion from ICD-9-CM to ICD-10-CM. Physicians should conduct annual examinations of patients and keep documenting the status of both chronic and acute conditions. Remember that HCC codes serve as payment multipliers.

Scenario 3: Earache

SCENARIO DETAILS

CHIEF COMPLAINT

- Right earache and ear pain

HISTORY

- A 20-year-old male patient who visits often is a full-time college student who started experiencing right-sided ear pain, noted 8/10 yesterday. However, these symptoms worsened, and acetaminophen didn't help to alleviate the pain. Luckily, we didn't notice any discharge, hearing loss, ringing/roaring, trauma, or recent barotrauma to the ear, including fever, sore throat, and cough today. Moreover, his previous URI was resolved with OTC medications in the past.

- Currently on his influenza, HPV, Tdap, and meningococcal immunizations

- The patient doesn't use tobacco, alcohol, or illicit drugs, and he is not exposed to secondhand smoke.

- He has been diagnosed with major depressive disorder with repeated episodes of mild severity and bipolar II disorder, while his current medications are aripiprazole and duloxetine.

- No known allergies

- 16-point review of systems negative apart from notations above

EXAM

- Healthy looking male, A&Ox3, calm, and cooperative

- Vital signs: BP: 130/78 HR: 70 bpm T: 99.8°F Wt: 235 lbs Ht: 5′ 10″

- ENT: Auricle and external canals normal bilaterally. Right ear: erythematous membrane bulging with loss of landmarks. Pharynx, teeth, and nose exam normal. No cervical adenopathy bilaterally

- Integumentary: Skin is flushed, warm, and dry without edema. Mucous membranes are moist.

- Respiratory: Lungs clear CTA with normal respiratory effort.

- Abdomen: Non-tender, no organomegaly

ASSESSMENT AND PLAN

- New onset AOM AD, suppurative, with pain unrelieved by acetaminophen

- Prescriptions: Amoxicillin for AOM; ibuprofen for pain

- Come back in one week if symptoms persist.

- Summary of ICD-10-CM impacts

CLINICAL DOCUMENTATION

- When diagnosing otitis media with ICD-9-CM, you should document items like acute, chronic, not specified as acute or chronic, nonsuppurative or suppurative, and with or without spontaneous rupture of the eardrum. To assign the correct code in ICD-10-CM, you should document additional features like the affected side (left, right, or bilateral) and indicate if it is a first-time occurrence or a repeated episode, as well as the previously mentioned details.

- In this fictional test case, we diagnosed this young male with bipolar II disorder. Do not report bipolar disorder unless it affects treatment at today's encounter. Don't report conditions that are not treated or that do not affect patient treatment.

CODING

ICD-9-CM DIAGNOSIS CODES

- 382.00 Acute suppurative otitis media without spontaneous rupture of the eardrum

ICD-10-CM DIAGNOSIS CODES

- H66.001 Acute suppurative otitis media without spontaneous rupture of the eardrum, right ear

OTHER IMPACTS

- No specific impact was noted.

Scenario 4: Anemia

SCENARIO DETAILS

CHIEF COMPLAINT

- Discuss laboratory results.

HISTORY

- Over a week ago, I examined a 38-year-old female patient, a regular visitor to our clinic, who has been experiencing decreased exercise tolerance and general malaise for the past four weeks, particularly during her daily aerobics class. During that visit, we ordered laboratory tests. Currently, she has been diagnosed with pale skin, weakness, and epigastric pain, which have remained unchanged since her last visit. Today's laboratory studies revealed the following results: HGB 8.5 gm/dL, HCT 27%, platelets 300,000/mm^3, reticulocytes 0.24%, MCV 75, serum iron 41 mcg/dL, serum ferritin 9 ng/ml, TIBC 457 mcg/dL, and a positive fecal occult blood test.

- For over three months, she kept taking esomeprazole to manage GERD with esophagitis, depending on over-the-counter antacids at night to relieve epigastric pain, as well as appropriate usage of ibuprofen to tackle headaches.

- Present pain is 0/10

- We need medical history for GERD, peptic ulcer, and pre-eclampsia with the last pregnancy.

- The last menstrual period (LMP) was two weeks ago, with a regular and unchanged flow over the past three months.

- She is married with three children ages 15, 12, and 1 year old.

- The patient doesn't use tobacco, alcohol, or illicit drugs.

- There are no known allergies.

- We couldn't find changes in the interval history and review of systems, unlike the previous encounter, which was eight days ago.

EXAM

- A healthy, well-groomed female who has good judgment and insight. Oriented X 3. She has good recent and remote memories as well as an adequate mood and affect.

- Vital signs: T 98.7°F, RR 18, BP: 118/75, standing 120/60, HR: 90

- HEENT: PERRLA

- Neck: Supple. No thyromegaly

- Lungs: Clear to auscultation with normal respiratory effort

- Cardiovascular: Normal rate and rhythm. No pedal edema

- Integumentary: Pale, clear of rashes and lesions, no ulcers. There is presence of early cheilosis.

- Rectal: No gross blood on exam one week ago, and stool sample results are seen above.

- Lymphatics: No lymphadenopathy

- Musculoskeletal: The patient had a good, stable walk.

ASSESSMENT AND PLAN

- Iron deficiency anemia was secondary to blood loss.

- Keep taking esomeprazole as prescribed.

- Substitute ibuprofen use with acetaminophen extra strength for headaches, according to the dosage instruction on the label.

- Prescribed iron sulfate supplements for a three-month trial and counseled the patient on the appropriate use of iron supplementation and its side effects.

- The patient should come back in one week for repeat laboratory studies.

SUMMARY OF ICD-10-CM IMPACTS

CLINICAL DOCUMENTATION

- In ICD-10-CM, gastro-esophageal reflux disease is distinguished by noting "with esophagitis" versus "without esophagitis." "With esophagitis" must be documented in the record.

CODING

ICD-9-CM DIAGNOSIS CODES

- 280.0 Iron deficiency anemia secondary to blood loss (chronic)

- 530.81 Disease, gastroesophageal reflux (GERD)

ICD-10-CM DIAGNOSIS CODES

- D50.0 Iron deficiency anemia secondary to blood loss (chronic)

- K21.0 Gastro-esophageal reflux disease with esophagitis

OTHER IMPACTS

- 530.11 Reflux esophagitis is not coded when GERD is coded in ICD-9-CM because 530.11 is an "excluded code" from 530.81 in ICD-9-CM, but it is a combination code in ICD-10-CM.

Step-by-Step Breakdown of Coding Complex Medical Cases

Coding complex medical cases isn't easy when you come across them, but you can still break down the process through a systematic approach. The following are the steps in the breakdown of coding complex medical cases:

Step 1: Review the medical documentation

Thoroughly evaluate the patient's medical records, i.e., the physician's notes, operative reports, diagnostic test results, and any other important documents, as well as understand the patient's medical condition, the procedures performed, and any complications or comorbidities.

Step 2: Identify the primary diagnosis

Determine what is responsible for the patient's encounter or hospitalization (i.e., a specific disease, injury, or symptom). You can obtain the primary diagnosis from the physician's assessment or the reason for the procedure.

Step 3: Identify secondary diagnoses and complications

You can identify any additional diagnoses to support the patient's condition, such as comorbidities, complications, or conditions that coexist with the primary diagnosis. Additional documentation to support the reporting of each secondary diagnosis should be performed.

Step 4: Assign appropriate diagnosis codes

When you understand the primary and secondary diagnoses, you can assign the proper diagnosis codes with the help of a standardized coding system such as the ICD-10-CM. Hence, find the specific codes that are related to each diagnosis for accuracy and specificity.

Step 5: Understand the procedures performed

Review the physician's notes and operative reports to discover the procedures performed during the patient's encounter. Then learn the details of each procedure, such as the specific techniques, instruments used, and any complications or extra procedures performed.

Step 6: Assign appropriate procedure codes

Assigning the right codes for each procedure performed can be done with a standardized coding system such as CPT or the International Classification of Diseases, 10th Revision, Procedure Coding System (ICD-10-PCS). Make sure the codes accurately reflect the details of the procedure in addition to any modifiers or additional services provided.

Step 7: Follow coding guidelines and rules

Consider the coding guidelines and rules provided by the coding system being used as they provide specific instructions for code assignment, sequencing, modifiers, and other coding conventions. Don't overlook the rules concerning primary and secondary diagnoses, procedure sequencing, and bundling or unbundling of services.

Step 8: Validate and double-check the codes

Evaluate the codes assigned for accuracy and completeness. After that, cross-reference the codes with the medical documentation to ensure alignment with the documented procedures and diagnoses. Finally, double-check for any errors or omissions in the code selection.

Step 9: Stay up-to-date with coding changes

Take note of the latest updates and changes in medical coding guidelines, coding systems, and regulatory requirements. Continue reviewing updates from organizations such as the American Medical Association (AMA), Centers for Medicare and Medicaid Services (CMS), and other important authorities.

Step 10: Seek clarification when needed

With ambiguous or incomplete documentation, consult the healthcare provider or physician to clarify the details because effective communication and collaboration with the medical team ensures accurate code assignment.

Note that coding complex medical cases means that you must have adequate knowledge of medical terminology, anatomy, and coding guidelines, so keep learning and refining your skills to code these cases effectively.

Detailed Examples of Coding Using Different Coding Systems

Many coding systems are used in the healthcare industry, for instance, the ICD-10-CM, CPT, and HCPCS. Below are detailed examples of coding using each of these systems:

1. ICD-10-CM:

You can use the ICD-10-CM to classify and code diagnoses and symptoms; it utilizes alphanumeric codes and provides a detailed range of codes for many medical conditions. Below is an example of ICD-10-CM coding:

- Diagnosis: Acute bronchitis

- ICD-10-CM Code: J20.9

Explanation: The code J20.9 represents acute bronchitis, unspecified. The "J" category represents diseases of the respiratory system, and the "20" subcategory represents acute bronchitis. The ".9" extension symbolizes an unspecified code.

2. CPT:

You can use the CPT codes to describe the medical procedures and services offered by healthcare professionals. The AMA manages these codes. Below is an example of CPT coding:

- Procedure: Evaluation and Management (E&M) visit

- CPT Code: 99213

Explanation: The CPT code 99213 represents an E&M visit at a regular physician's office. Physicians use these visits for a detailed history and examination and for medical decision-making for evaluating a patient's condition, discussing treatment options, and managing their care.

3. HCPCS:

You can use the HCPCS codes to identify and bill medical supplies, durable medical equipment (DME), prosthetics, orthotics, and other healthcare services. Below is an example of HCPCS coding:

- Service: Urinary catheter, two-way Foley

- HCPCS Code: A4352

Explanation: The HCPCS code A4352 is assigned to a two-way Foley urinary catheter. Use this code to detect and bill the specific type of catheter used in the procedure.

Note that these are just examples, and medical coding has lots of codes and guidelines. The specific codes and guidelines applicable to a certain case may be different based on factors such as the patient's condition, the type of service provided, and the healthcare setting. As a medical coder, you should be trained to use coding manuals and guidelines to assign codes accurately.

Key Takeaways

- Medical coding helps you to document and communicate patient diagnoses, procedures, and treatments accurately.

- The practical exercises in this chapter use real-world coding scenarios and enable critical thinking.

- The detailed breakdowns of complex cases let you break down complex scenarios with the required tools for successful coding.

- The detailed coding examples using different coding systems (e.g., ICD-10-CM, CPT, HCPCS) help you learn how to translate medical documentation into accurate codes.

- You can code common medical scenarios by documenting specific pain locations, distinguishing alcohol-related disorders, and offering more specific codes for abdominal tenderness.

- You need the given scenarios for diagnosis codes from both ICD-9-CM and ICD-10-CM coding systems.

- In your clinical documentation, you should document the purpose of the encounter, cases of the patient stopping their medication, and specific features of conditions such as their acuteness, chronicity, or suppurative nature.

- You may experience various impacts and considerations in specific scenarios, such as Medicare Advantage risk adjustment plans or the relevance of preventative health incentives for annual exams.

There is much to learn before you can obtain your first job as a medical biller and coder, so check out the next chapter.

CHAPTER 6: BREAKING INTO THE INDUSTRY

This chapter teaches practical tips and strategies for those who want to break into the industry. You'll learn how to land your first job as a medical coder and overcome the common challenge of not having enough experience. We'll also discuss why you need to participate in networking, join professional associations, and build a portfolio to enhance your chances of finding job opportunities. So apply the insights in this chapter to navigate the industry, establish your presence, and begin a successful career as a medical coder.

Tips for Landing Your First Job

Check out the following tips to land your first job.

1. Join a Professional Association

Professional associations usually help candidates to get their first jobs as well as provide many additional benefits for their careers, including:

- Continuing education opportunities

- Networking events

- Job opportunities

- Specialty certifications

- Career training resources

- Up-to-date career news and industry changes

Below are two major professional associations for medical coders and billers:

a. The American Association of Professional Coders (AAPC)

AAPC is the largest training and credentialing coding association in the world and has more than 190,000 members worldwide. This organization provides updated medical coding and billing industry resources, classes on honing your work skills, and annual healthcare conferences.

b. American Health Information Management Association (AHIMA)

AHIMA is a nonprofit organization for health information professionals. The AHIMA website claims the organization is "the leading authority on health information." Members of AHIMA enjoy several benefits, including receiving updates on industry news, networking opportunities, professional development, and career advice.

2. Get Certified as a CPC/CPC-A

Being a certified professional coder, or CPC, is another effective way to beat your competitors and enhance your job prospects. Certification as a CPC enables you to handle medical billing and coding claims, payments, insurance, and patient billing communication.

Since certifications and education are what employers first consider when reviewing candidates, certification proves that you have initiative and are committed to the job you are interviewing for.

Medical offices and institutions worldwide see medical billing and coding certifications as the universally accepted "gold standard." Today, the American Academy of Professional Coders, or AAPC, has certified more than 159,000 healthcare workers.

3. Become an Office or Front Desk Staff in a Healthcare Facility

Front desk receptionists in a healthcare facility can gain valuable experience in the field, increasing your chances of becoming a medical coder or biller. Prove your expertise as a front desk receptionist to stay informed about vacant medical or coding positions by maintaining a good relationship with the hiring manager. This will increase your chances of securing an interview.

4. Work with a Temp Agency

Temporary, or temp, employment agencies are good for both the employer and the employee. The employer can easily hire the right staff without advertising the position and passing through the hurdles of interviewing many candidates. The employee is hired through a contract for a short period that typically lasts for six months or less. Agencies vet prospective employees, helping to ensure a good fit for both the employer and the employee.

Temp agencies receive requests from all kinds of facilities and often know of job openings that cannot be found elsewhere. Therefore, a temp agency can quickly give you valuable work experience to start earning money from your medical billing and coding job.

Note that some temporary employers may offer a temp-to-hire position. This arrangement allows temporary employees who have met or exceeded expectations during the contract period the opportunity to progress into a full-time position with the company.

5. Volunteer

Volunteering also helps aspiring medical billers and coders in two ways. First, it lets you fill in your résumé gaps, particularly if you prefer to work for a long time. Second, volunteering in a healthcare facility you are interested in usually gives you direct access to hiring managers.

6. Job Shadow

At times, shadowing a friend or family member working in the medical and coding industry can get you closer in your pursuit of a new job.

Job shadowing helps you understand that position. Since you already know the person you are shadowing, it is easier to understand the business. So if you can shadow someone in the industry, ask as many questions as possible to increase your knowledge.

This strategy makes employers recognize that you are on a job hunt and will surely be an asset to their team. Hand over your résumé to the hiring manager for perusal when you get the chance.

7. Start with an Internship

An internship gives you hands-on work experience in a setting where you will end up working. Note that not all internships are paid, and if you are paid, you'll get much less than what you would earn as a staff member of the organization. However, there are several benefits of doing an internship:

- You will have access to on-the-job networking.

- You will get valuable work experience to add to your résumé and beat your competitors.

- You will have the chance to put your education into action and hone your skills.

- You can progress into a new job after your internship ends.

8. Work as a Medical Records Clerk

As a medical records clerk, you can manage patient files within a healthcare facility and work with some of the same healthcare facilities that also hire medical billers and coders. Moreover, there's an opportunity to work in medical records during your medical coding and billing education to get the upper hand on your fellow graduates!

You Can Do This!

Hustling and commitment can help you get your first medical billing and coding job. However, being focused and implementing one or more of the above methods will make you a medical biller and coder before you realize it. Good luck to you on your job search!

Ten Jobs That You Can Do with a Medical Billing and Coding Certificate

You will get several job opportunities with a certificate in medical billing and coding because there are various fields available. Below is a list of 10 jobs you can do with a certificate for medical billing and coding:

1. Medical biller

National average salary: $31,287 per year

Primary duties: As a medical biller, you submit a coded transcript that has a summary of a patient's visit to their insurance company to file a claim. Medical billers collaborate with medical coders who create the medical coding to translate information through specialty software and send it to the insurance company for review. Medical billers act as an intermediary between insurance companies, healthcare providers, and patients, so they usually possess more knowledge of both insurance and healthcare. Some of their duties are to review patient bills, set up payment plans, and appeal dismissed claims.

2. Medical records technician

National average salary: $38,482 per year

Primary duties: A medical records technician ensures the accuracy of a patient's medical records, which will be used by a medical coder to create the needed codes for insurance claims. They track and update a patient's medical history, past claims, treatments, and other confidential information so that healthcare providers and their patients receive the proper reimbursement from insurance carriers. They are also responsible for transcribing these records into codes that comply with the appropriate coding guidelines and policies.

3. Billing analyst

National average salary: $38,676 per year

Primary duties: A billing analyst ensures a patient is charged the correct amount on their bill and can also provide customer support by communicating with customers directly, answering their queries, and managing their issues. In addition, billing analysts examine invoices and correct any inconsistencies by seeking clarification from other departments or an insurance carrier. Furthermore, they evaluate the existing billing procedures and software as well as provide feedback to management on potential enhancements.

4. Medical collector

National average salary: $38,811 per year

Primary duties: Medical collectors receive overdue payments from patients for their medical services like routine visits, hospitalizations and overnight stays, surgeries, and other forms of treatment. They can work directly for a medical facility as in-house collectors or collection agencies. Medical collectors communicate with patients and provide alternative methods of payment to assist patients who can't pay immediately.

5. Medical records coordinator

National average salary: $44,587 per year

Primary duties: Medical records coordinators are senior-level medical professionals who manage and maintain confidential patient records. They collaborate with doctors, nurses, and other medical staff members to verify that they're accurately recording, organizing, and maintaining secure data. These coordinators also maintain the specialty software for managing a patient's medical data and information. They offer patient records to doctors and nurses and secure any confidential information in the records.

6. Coding Specialist

National average salary: $48,224 per year

Primary duties: A coding specialist creates medical coding that contains the summary of a patient's visit so that a medical biller can submit an insurance claim. These codes are used to record information such as a patient's symptoms and diagnosis, prescribed medications, therapies, surgeries, and other required treatments. They collaborate with doctors, medical assistants, and medical billers to ensure an accurately transcribed patient's visit summary and other information and prevent insurance claim discrepancies.

7. Coding educator

National average salary: $55,628 per year

Primary duties: A coding educator teaches students everything they should know about coding by creating a curriculum, crafting lesson plans, and offering engaging presentations. They also participate in coding and reimbursement meetings as well as other relevant events, to remain updated on current trends and information. Lastly, they create training materials like study guides and handbooks to help students complete their courses.

8. Coding auditor

National average salary: $61,016 per year

Primary duties: A coding auditor oversees coding operations to confirm that the information is accurately transcribed to ensure all medical bills are accurate for a patient. Coding auditors also record regular coding mistakes and report them to management. They support medical coders by offering feedback on their performances when needed, educating and training them with useful tips and techniques to get better at coding.

9. Lawyer

National average salary: $74,205 per year

Primary duties: A lawyer who operates in the medical law industry assists clients who need help in handling billing fraud cases. For instance, a lawyer may advocate for a client in a case where a specific medical code is deliberately entered incorrectly to add or remove a service or treatment from a patient's visit summary. Lawyers review medical documents, files, and bills related to a medical lawsuit.

10. Clinical informaticists

National average salary: $83,979 per year

Primary duties: A clinical informaticist uses information technologies like data entry software and visual image storage systems to help doctors offer optimal treatment for patients. Informaticists also teach staff about using specialized software and systems. They are IT specialists who troubleshoot, install, and integrate new systems across various departments to improve their functionalities. They also enhance the workflow by evaluating existing software and systems and making needed changes.

Note: Salary figures mentioned are national average salaries and may differ based on various factors, including experience, location, and employer.

Networking and Professional Associations

In this section, you'll learn how to network and which professional associations are relevant to a medical biller and coder.

Networking

Professional networking may include in-person or online contacts, and it helps billing and coding program graduates to improve their career development via connections in the field as well as grow employment prospects. Conferences and seminars are networking events that can help graduates find mentors and share knowledge and resources within the industry, including identifying new job opportunities.

LinkedIn is an online professional networking website that can help medical billing and coding graduates establish virtual connections through existing professional relationships. You must possess good interpersonal skills, confidence in your expertise, and the will to take moderate risks to advance your career in any type of setting for professional networking to take place.

Networking efforts usually focus on professional relationships; however, they can also foster connections for people working in similar fields to find commonalities in their personal lives. These more personalized contacts can lead to long-term, symbiotic relationships between professionals in medical billing and coding. Networking is also great for people without much experience in the field to gain entry, especially medical billing and coding graduates desiring to explore various work environments.

Networking Tips in Medical Billing and Coding

- Take Notes: After establishing a strong professional network connection, document it for future reference. Use a few minutes to record their contact information, their usefulness to you, and any other key points worth remembering about the interaction after the conversation.

- Ask Questions: Although sharing your personal life or professional goals is important, give the other party in a networking conversation a listening ear. Ask thoughtful questions about their career path or the particulars of their current job.

- Share Unnecessary Connections with Others: You might meet people who are not valuable to you in professional networking.

119

However, they could be useful to your colleagues, so share the contact's information with them. They might also connect you to such people in the future.

- Take Note of Your Body Language: Your self-confidence isn't just about how you move your feet, blink, or swallow but also includes your body language and your behavior in professional situations. Remember to smile, keep an upright posture while standing or sitting, and greet others by confidently shaking their hands.

- Conduct Research Beforehand: You should do some research on the work and career paths of the speakers and other attendees you want to connect with before attending any professional networking event. Then ask meaningful questions and show your familiarity with their work for longer-lasting and more relevant professional relationships.

Dos and Don'ts for Networking Events:

Dos:

- Set achievable goals at networking events.

- Dress professionally.

- Take business cards to exchange contact information.

- Be concise and communicate relevant information effectively.

120

- Follow up with your connections after the event.

Don'ts:

- Focus more on distributing paper résumés than in-person conversations for more effective networking.

- Use a shotgun approach and try to meet as many people as possible without building meaningful connections.

- Interrupt or talk over others; instead, listen actively and show respect for others' contributions.

- Be intimidated by others' credentials or experience; contribute to the conversation confidently.

- Neglect to follow up on connections; value their potential contribution to your career and maintain professional relationships.

Professional Associations

The following are professional associations to consider as medical billers and coders:

- American Academy of Professional Coders (AAPC): Offers education and certification for professional medical coders with links to local chapters.

- American Health Information Management Association (AHIMA): Offers a career/job bank, ongoing educational opportunities, certification information, and an extensive section on coding and the existing coding system.

- Medical Association of Billers (MAB): MAB is an international support organization that offers training in the ICD and CPT. This site also offers a forum for discussing issues and asking questions, as well as information on dental billing and coding.

- Professional Association of Healthcare Coding Specialists (PAHCS): PAHCS is a communications network and member support system that keeps enhancing the compliance, documentation, and reimbursement capabilities of healthcare coders.

Building a Portfolio and Gaining Experience

Building a portfolio and gaining experience in medical billing and coding is easy with the following steps:

1. Education and Certification: Complete a reputable medical billing and coding program or online course, as well as obtain certifications like the CPC or CCS.

2. Volunteering or Internships: Volunteer or become an intern in healthcare facilities or medical billing companies to gain hands-on experience and understand coding and billing processes.

3. Practice Coding Exercises: Continuously practice coding exercises online or through coding books to enhance skills and proficiency in managing diverse coding scenarios.

4. Build a Coding Portfolio: Showcase your skills and expertise by adding examples of medical records, coding assignments, and significant projects in a professional portfolio to show potential employers or clients.

5. Join Professional Associations: Join associations such as the AAPC or the AHIMA to gain resources, networking, and industry updates.

6. Seek Entry-Level Positions: Apply for entry-level positions to showcase your education, certifications, and practical experience earned through volunteering or internships.

7. Continuous Learning: Stay updated with industry changes via ongoing education programs, workshops, and conferences, as well as consider advanced certifications or specialization to increase your expertise.

Comply with these steps and regularly improve your knowledge and skills to build a solid foundation and gain more success in this field.

Key Takeaways

- Landing your first job as a medical coder isn't easy, but perseverance and the right strategies can help.

- Join a professional association such as the AAPC or the AHIMA to get networking opportunities, career resources, and job leads.

- Work to become certified as a CPC/CPC-A to enhance your job prospects and showcase your commitment to the field.

- You need experience in the healthcare industry, even in noncoding roles as a front desk receptionist or medical records clerk, to progress into a coding position.

- When you work with a temp agency, you'll gain valuable work experience and eventually get a permanent job.

- Volunteering in healthcare facilities fills gaps in your résumé and connects you with hiring managers.

- Job shadowing someone in the industry provides more knowledge of the field and builds relationships with potential employers.

- Being an intern gives you hands-on experience in the same setting you'll be working in, and sometimes you can access full-time positions.

- You will gain valuable experience as a medical records clerk and understand the healthcare environment.

- Medical billing and coding certification gives you access to various job opportunities as a medical biller, medical records technician, billing analyst, medical collector, coding specialist, coding educator, coding auditor, a lawyer specializing in medical law, or clinical informatics.

- Network for career development in medical billing and coding, using both in-person and online networking to create connections and find mentors and job opportunities.

- You'll get valuable resources, education, certification information, and networking opportunities as a medical biller and coder from associations such as AAPC, AHIMA, MAB, and PAHCS.

- You can build a portfolio and gain experience through education, certification, internships, volunteering, and taking on roles such as medical records clerk.

You've learned how to break into the industry and be successful; now, you need to learn how to thrive in your career. Go to the next chapter for more information.

CHAPTER 7: THRIVING IN YOUR NEW CAREER

It is not news that the medical coding industry is an ever-changing one. As such, you have to learn to position yourself to be properly equipped to adjust to whatever the industry brings your way as a medical biller and coder. In addition to this, you will also need to learn how to be fast-paced in what you do while still ensuring that you are accurate, and this is exactly what this chapter will help you achieve. This chapter will also go a step further into how to navigate the challenges that are peculiar to the industry.

Keeping Up with Industry Changes and Ongoing Education

The healthcare industry, like any other industry, is going to experience a series of evolutions over time. It is crucial that in order to stay relevant within the industry, you are updated with the latest information regarding medical billing and coding. This will not only help you to develop your knowledge in the sphere but also make you able to adapt to the latest updates and development. Below are a few tips on what to do to stay informed on the latest updates and changes in the medical billing and coding industry:

- The first step to take when you are seeking to thrive in your career as a medical biller and coder is to make sure that you are up-to-date with the international classification of diseases database.
- Furthermore, you must also ensure that you engage in research that will enlighten you on the latest trends and developments that

the industry experiences. For example, there have been recent technologies that have characterized changes within the industry. Some of these changes are cloud practice management platforms, the medical Internet of things, and electronic health records.

In addition to the aforementioned changes, there have been changes in the regulations of privacy, such as HIPAA and the payment card industry data security standard (PCI-DSS), that have had a profound impact on the way medical billers and coders treat the patients' personal identifiable information (PII) and payment details. Staying informed on these updates helps you ensure that your practice is up to speed and acceptable.

- Another way that you can thrive in your career as a medical coder and biller is to become a member of professional bodies and network with individuals who have already made headway in the field. For example, you can choose to be a member of the American Academy of Professional Coders or American Health Information Management. These bodies provide numerous materials in order for their members to remain current with updates relating to medical billing and coding. Also, subscribing to the industries' newsletters and actively participating in forums and discussions can help you become informed on new updates.

- The role of professional certifications in this discourse cannot be overstated. For example, certifications like RHIT, HRHIA, and CPC-P from AHIMA and AAPC may help you prepare to pursue opportunities like a supervisory or management role in medical billing and coding. You can also decide to improve your skills in health information management or healthcare administration and services to enhance your career choices.

If you are considering taking professional courses, it is important for you to explore online platforms that avail you the opportunity to do so. This is so that you can easily navigate through your studies and continue your work schedule as well.

Balancing Speed and Accuracy

As we noted earlier, speed and accuracy are two effective skills required in the industry. While the idea of embracing speed in your work and still being accurate may seem like a difficult task, it is important to know that it is not an impossible one to embark on. In order to master the art of speed and accuracy on the job, the following tips are recommended:

- Ensure that you are properly equipped with the foundational knowledge of medical coding and billing. Understanding the peculiarities of the profession will improve your chances of being able to carry it out seamlessly. Be properly equipped with knowledge of guidelines such as the international classification of disease codes and current procedural terminology.
- The electronic health record revolutionized the medical coding process, bringing it into the digital age. The EHR is still the key

to medical coding, but other technologies are emerging to improve quality and accuracy.

Software products such as computer-assisted code (CAC) can be used to analyze documents in order to determine the correct medical codes. These solutions can speed up the process while still ensuring accuracy.

- Take advantage of coding resources available to you on the internet, such as coding software, manuals, and other tools. These materials offer guidance and various tips that help you to code at a quick pace and with more accuracy.

- Medical coding requires a great level of concentration. You must ensure that while on the job, you pay keen attention to the details. Try as much as you can to minimize the level of your distraction. If possible, ensure that your workspace is one that allows you to give maximum attention to coding. This will help you maintain a high level of accuracy while on the job.

- Take time out to create templates for coding processes and scenarios that you believe will be continuous and progressive. This action will no doubt save a great deal of time by proffering a certain framework that you can utilize rather than starting from scratch every single time.

- Making a culture of time management will also improve your speed, accuracy, and productivity on the job. Time management brings balance to speed and accuracy. Set reasonable time frames to carry out certain coding tasks. Also, ensure that you always prioritize more important assignments, and whenever you are confronted with complex tasks, you assign a reasonable time frame for them.

- If you come across ambiguous or unclear documentation, it is best to seek clarification from the healthcare provider. Clear communication enables accurate coding and prevents delays or errors.

- Finally, it is also very important that you carry out regular audits and reviews of your coding work to identify any patterns of errors or areas that need improvement. Learning from mistakes and regularly improving your coding skills will promote both speed and accuracy.

Ensure that speed is never prioritized over accuracy in medical billing and coding. First, focus on the accuracy of the coding because errors can yield denial of claims, reimbursement delays, or even legal issues. Therefore, with practice, experience, and regular improvement, you can attain a balance between speed and accuracy in your coding processes.

Dealing with Common Challenges and How to Overcome Them

While pursuing a career in medical billing and coding might be challenging, every obstacle along the way improves your expertise. Below are the top seven challenges that medical billing and coding experts should address and how they affect their professional growth.

1. Medical Information Is under Medical Privacy Laws

You should know by now that medical coding as a profession entails handling sensitive data, and this requires that you comply with medical privacy laws like HIPAA privacy security rules or the Health Information Technology for Economic and Clinical Health (HITECH) Act. As a professional, you must ensure that while you code, you take into consideration the national standards that apply to safeguarding a patient's health information. Complying with privacy laws is essential; hence, you must ensure that you adhere strictly to the guidelines.

Since the law strictly regulates information in medical records, as an expert, you should learn about legal matters related to your work. You must ensure full confidentiality to secure patient privacy, making your job one of great responsibility and demanding careful attention to all details.

2. Understanding Medical Billing and Coding Systems

As part of medical billing and coding education, students must learn standard systems. Electronic medical records (EMR) and electronic health records (EHR) are the most common software among these. Although they both contain digitized versions, the differences are noticeable. The EMR is a digital version of a chart for a single healthcare facility. However, the EHR contains a more comprehensive picture of the patient's health.

Just like anything else, EMR and EHR are no exceptions to the rule that nothing is perfect. Both have their own downsides. Both systems require some time to master and rely on third-party support. It is vital that the system runs smoothly, so it is essential to update it frequently. Another disadvantage of making use of electronic health records software is the possibility of data breaches. Although they are less common than other security breaches, they can have serious consequences for patients and health professionals.

There are other downsides to the system. Transferring data from EMRs to other practices can be stressful. EHR systems are also volatile and can be hacked.

3. Possible Errors When Extracting Data from Medical Records

There are chances that in the process of extracting data from medical records, certain errors surface. These errors range from typographical errors to reporting unlisted codes without documentation. Since every symbol matters, knowing and offering valid procedure codes is relevant. However, errors in the medical billing process could be associated with missing or inaccurate information.

For example, issuing duplicate bills, creating mismatched invoices, or not providing enough details to support a claim are all errors that can create havoc in the billing and coding system. As mentioned in Chapter 3 under "Ethical Considerations and the Importance of Accuracy," upcoding is another bad practice that happens when a health service or treatment bill is more costly than it should have been. It usually results from referring to a diagnosis or condition that is more severe than the actual one.

4. Technical Updates in Medical Billing and Coding

The ever-changing nature of medical codes may sometimes result in some errors. Every year, certain codes are either amended or changed. One challenge you most likely will encounter is trying to stay updated with these trends. Apparently, the most appropriate way to overcome technical updates in medical billing and coding is to ensure that you utilize the available channels to keep informed when there is a change or revision in the system.

5. Medical Billing and Coding Includes Third-Parties

The profession requires that there is regular if not frequent communication between the parties involved, such as insurance companies, government agencies, health maintenance organizations, and employers. The interdependent nature of the profession requires that you have a reasonable extent of patience, politeness, and persistence as well. The best way to ensure that you relate with the numerous parties involved is to develop interpersonal relationship traits. Luckily, anyone who is a good listener and good communicator will be unlikely to encounter any problems relating to other individuals.

6. Pandemic Changes for Medical Billers and Coders

The unpredictable nature of the world may require that a medical biller and coder work excessive hours. During the recent pandemic that swept the whole world like a tornado, institutions employing medical billers and coders began to operate 24/7 with shifts that were quite different than they were before the pandemic. After the COVID-19 outbreak, new standards were set, with working remotely as one of them. Today, professionals can perform their duties remotely, which might become a successful practice in the future.

Furthermore, new COVID-19 coding guidelines were released. As discussed above, they were a quick response to the unfolding crisis. Therefore, medical billing and coding professionals should easily adapt to any updates coming into force.

7. Medical Billing and Coding Certification Renewal

Like any other health professionals, medical billers and coders have to renew their professional certifications intermittently. Renowned organizations all expect members to renew their certifications by completing ongoing education units and paying a renewal fee. Your continuous dedication demonstrated by maintaining certification shows you are a lifelong learner and boosts your employability. Pursuing the amazing career opportunities in medical billing and coding across the US is worthwhile. A job in medical billing and coding will particularly benefit you in the state of NJ, where the salaries of all allied health specialists are highly profitable.

Key Takeaways

- Keep up-to-date with the latest medical billing and coding trends, industry regulations, and HIPAA/PCI-DSS.
- Subscribe to professional newsletters and attend conferences in order to keep informed.
- Use coding resources and develop a solid base in medical coding.
- Use templates, standard processes, and time management.
- Ask for clarification when necessary and audit your work regularly.
- Stay up-to-date with the latest technical developments, communicate with third parties, and adapt to changing conditions such as pandemics.
- Certification shows that you are committed to lifelong learning, and it increases your employability.
- Medical billers and coders can earn a lot of money, especially in states such as NJ, where allied health specialists are paid well.

- There are many ways to maximize your income after you learn how to succeed in your medical billing career. The next chapter will tell you how to do that.

CHAPTER 8: MAXIMIZING YOUR EARNINGS

Anyone who engages in any sort of profession knows that there is a need to make the most of their finances. This is what is referred to as the act of maximizing your earnings. The purpose of this chapter is to give you a perspective on how to make the best of your earnings. This chapter emphasizes the need to be a specialist in the medical coding profession as well as how to get additional certifications in the process.

Strategies for Increasing Your Income

There is nothing more satisfying than doing what you love with ease and making a good deal of money from it. No one ever gets tired of making more money. Below are various strategies that you can take advantage of to increase your income as a medical biller and coder:

1. Earn More Certifications: Salary surveys have repeatedly proven that having multiple certifications will lead an employer to understand your worth and passion for the job, and it increases your competency in your work. Therefore, there is a higher probability that your pay increases when you are certified by reputable platforms.

2. Try Remote Coding Opportunities: The more opportunities you have to work jobs, the higher your chances of earning more. One way to do this is to try remote coding jobs. You can apply online for different companies and on different platforms to make more money aside from your regular job.

3. Gain Experience and Face Challenges: Keep learning even when you are on the job and increase your expertise in the field. Also, ensure that you are never too scared to take up a challenge, regardless of how daunting it may seem. As the popular saying goes, challenges are blessings in disguise. When an employer sees how you have continuously navigated challenges, chances are that he or she will find you competent and increase your salary.

4. Develop Additional Skills: Aside from gaining multiple credentials in medical billing and coding, you can also choose to learn other relevant skills like Excel or PowerPoint to keep you ahead of your competition. The company might find your additional competencies beneficial and increase your pay instead of hiring someone else to fill another position. This makes you valuable to your team.

The Value of Specialization and Additional Certifications

Specializing and acquiring additional certifications in medical billing and coding offers several valuable benefits, including the following points listed below.

1. Increases Expertise: When you choose to stay focused on a particular niche, you are more likely to increase the level of your expertise in it. This is because you undoubtedly pay undivided attention to your selected niche. Hence, put a concerted effort into developing yourself in that field.

2. Competitive Advantage: Employers prefer candidates with specialized skills and certifications, giving you a competitive edge in the job market.

3. Profitability Increases: Your profitability level increases significantly when you are specialized. This is due to the increased demand of employers for individuals with higher expertise.

4. Career Advancement Opportunities: Specializations and certifications can open doors to higher-level positions and roles with more responsibility.

5. Staying Up-to-Date: Being specialized and gaining certificates avail you the opportunity to receive regular details about the trends in the industry, which is a much-needed prerequisite for your growth as a medical coder and biller.

By specializing and obtaining additional certifications, you enhance your skills, marketability, and earning potential while demonstrating your commitment to professional growth and providing high-quality healthcare services.

Negotiating Pay And Benefits

When negotiating pay and benefits in medical billing and coding:

1. Research Salary and Benefits: Gather information on industry standards and salary ranges to establish a benchmark for negotiation.

2. Highlight Your Value: Emphasize your skills, experience, and certifications and how your expertise can benefit the organization.

3. Prepare a Compelling Case: Showcase your achievements and demonstrate how your contributions have positively impacted previous employers.

4. Be Assertive and Confident: Approach negotiations with confidence, clearly expressing your expectations.

5. Consider the Total Compensation Package: Evaluate the entire compensation package, including benefits like healthcare coverage, retirement plans, and professional development opportunities.

Key Takeaways

- Gain multiple credentials to boost your competency and worth, resulting in higher salaries.

- Consider remote coding opportunities to supplement your income and expand your job options.

- Gain experience and face challenges to show competence and earn more salary.

- Develop additional skills beyond medical billing and coding to boost your worth to the company.

- Specialize and earn additional certifications to improve your expertise and stand out from generalists.

- Specializations and certifications offer a competitive advantage, higher earning potential, and career advancement opportunities.

- Specialized certifications prove your expertise and enhance your professional reputation.

- Negotiate pay and benefits by researching industry standards, outlining your value, and preparing a compelling case.

CHAPTER 9: BUILDING A LONG-TERM CAREER

Now that you're enlightened about your profession, you are ready to begin considering how to build a long-term career in medical billing and coding. In this chapter, we'll discuss career progression in medical billing and coding and move on to explore the various available opportunities for leadership and teaching in medical billing and coding. Finally, we'll also delve into the credentials required for starting your business.

Career Progression in Medical Billing and Coding

As stated previously, medical billing and coding is a career path that offers flexibility. It provides diverse opportunities for growth and advancement. Typically, the usual progression from the onset is that a person entering fresh into the field will most likely start out serving in an entry-level position. Most professionals begin their careers working as medical billing and coding specialists. People who occupy this position assign codes to diagnoses and procedures, process insurance claims, and manage patient billing. Entry-level positions regularly require a certificate or diploma in medical coding and billing.

After a person starts out in the industry, the desire to begin to explore more opportunities may surface. This desire is most likely going to prompt one into pursuing certifications recognized within the industry which will, in turn, undoubtedly improve career prospects. By now, you should know that the most popular certification in this field is the CPC credential provided by the AAPC. Attaining this certification demonstrates proficiency in coding systems like CPT, ICD, and HCPCS.

After gaining experience comes the need to specialize in a specific niche within the industry; this is what most professionals opt for next as they journey through this career path. Specializations can involve coding for certain medical specialties such as cardiology, orthopedics, or oncology. Specialized coders regularly earn higher salaries and have more career opportunities.

With many years of experience and a number of recognized certifications, you may then have the opportunity to take on a role as a team leader or in a supervisory position. These roles will enable you to oversee a team of medical coders and billers, offer guidance, and ensure accurate and timely coding and billing processes.

Another option available to you as you progress in your career that you may wish to consider is working in roles associated with audits and compliance. The major functions carried out within these roles are to review medical coding to ensure that the codes are accurate and also comply with established regulations both at the industry level and in the wider spectrum. Auditors identify coding errors, ensure adequate documentation, and reduce potential fraud and abuse.

The opportunity to work as an RCM professional is also another viable option. An RCM professional basically focuses on enhancing the financial performance of healthcare organizations by streamlining billing processes, managing denials and appeals, and improving strategies for reimbursement.

In addition to the aforementioned steps, one of the top roles that may open up to you as you pursue excellence in your practice is a managerial or administrative role. This role is basically a result of many years of experience and veritable leadership within the industry. Functions of these positions include overseeing billing and coding departments, setting policies, managing budgets, and working with other healthcare stakeholders to enhance revenue and compliance.

Finally, experienced professionals can become consultants or start their own independent coding and billing businesses. This path enables you to provide expertise and guidance to healthcare organizations, conduct audits, provide training, or even develop coding and billing software solutions.

Remember that career progression can differ based on factors like education, certifications, work experience, and the job market in your region. Ongoing learning, staying updated with industry changes, networking, and professional development activities can greatly enhance your career growth in medical billing and coding.

Opportunities for Leadership and Teaching

If you're passionate about impacting people with your skill, then this should be exciting to you. There are also opportunities within the industry that allow you to teach or mentor people about what you know from your experience working in the industry. Below are a few opportunities you could explore:

- Educational Institutions: There are organizations devoted to training people in the medical billing and coding industry. You can apply for positions as an instructor or program coordinator in vocational schools, community colleges, or universities that provide medical billing and coding programs.

- Moving further, you can become a member of organizations that offer specialized training and certification programs for medical billers and coders. You can work as a trainer or instructor within these organizations.

- You can also choose to join consultation firms. You can be a consultant for building startups as well as executive best practices.

- It is also possible that you can become a member of professional associations such as the AAPC or the Healthcare Information and Management Systems Society (HIMSS). Participate as a speaker or instructor in their workshops and educational events.

- You can also decide to train young people in the industry via online platforms. This will even grant you the opportunity to move further in what you do. You may choose to create relevant materials and offer them for sale to aid the pursuits of young enthusiasts in the industry. You can also opt to be a teacher on e-learning platforms and offer your services by providing courses.

- Continuing Education Programs: Create and provide ongoing education programs for healthcare organizations and medical billing and coding associations.

Obtaining needed certifications like the CPC credential and gaining expertise in certain areas, such as ICD-10 or electronic health records, can boost your chances of finding leadership and teaching roles.

The Potential for Starting Your Own Business

There is a huge potential for you to start your own business in the industry, and the most surprising part is that you do not necessarily need a great deal of capital. The status of the world today allows you to build a community without having physical contact with people. What this means is that you can begin your business carrying out your duties from the comfort of your home. There are industries that subscribe to the idea of outsourcing medical coding and billing functions to a third party, and if you do not have the resources to start out on a large scale, this is something you may wish to consider. Before you begin making a website design, it is highly advisable that you consult local healthcare providers to give you answers to these questions and equip yourself with the right knowledge.

- Do they do their billing in-house or outsource it?

- Does the outside coding company manage all the bills or just some of them?

- How many patients do they bill daily?

If the volume of patients is low or the market for billing services is saturated, it might be unwise to start a medical billing business. However, if you discern a need in your market area, 360Connect noted that it would cost you at least $1,000 to start from scratch. You'll need medical billing software, a reliable computer, reliable internet, a backup system, and money for tech support and repair.

It's essential to choose the right billing software. Although cost is a factor, the Nurse.org website says you should go for the most reliable, dependable software affordable. Also, consider ease of use, mobile options, and compatibility with related tasks.

AAPC recommends that you begin by enrolling in a medical billing or coding course at a university or online. The completion of a certification course and passing the test will enhance your credibility. You should also have experience as a coder in a billing department or for a well-established company. You will gain confidence, and you'll realize how much you love the job. You do not want to invest your resources in starting a medical billing company only to learn later that you don't like the work.

You can launch your business once you have everything in place—certifications, training, experience, and consulting with local healthcare providers. Your business will be successful if you adhere to a strict production schedule. You will be asked to code and charge for a certain number of procedures per day by your clients. Auditors will check your work to ensure it is accurate and complete.

Coders who are not certified earn an average of $47,200 per year. The AAPC reported that certification increases your income to an average of $61,917. The location, your education and training, and your credentials determine if you will earn more or less than the average.

Key Takeaways

- Medical billing and coding provide career progression opportunities.

- Entry-level positions as specialists are common and require certification or a diploma.

- Pursuing certifications such as CPC enhances career prospects.

- Specializing in certain areas of coding results in higher salaries and more opportunities.

- Progression can involve roles as team leaders, auditors, managers, and consultants.

- Leadership and teaching opportunities exist in educational institutions, training organizations, consulting firms, and associations.

- Starting a medical billing and coding business requires market research and a relatively modest investment.

- Choose reliable billing software and ensure you have the necessary training, certification, and experience.

- Successful businesses meet production schedules, ensure accurate coding, and undergo audits.

- Certification increases income potential, with certified coders earning an average of $61,917.

Congratulations, you have completed this journey of medical billing and coding, and you can check out the next chapter for a good overview of everything.

CONCLUSION: YOUR REWARDING CAREER IN MEDICAL BILLING AND CODING

There are amazing benefits that come with choosing the medical billing and coding industry as your career path. This benefit cuts across both your personal and professional development. This book has extensively discussed the need for in-depth knowledge of the industry, from understanding the key roles and responsibilities of medical billers and coders to exploring several coding systems.

Developing essential skills like analytical thinking, attention to detail, and proficiency with technology and software can help you succeed in this industry. Obtaining the required education and certifications will improve your expertise and credibility and prepare you for success.

Once you enter the industry, note that networking, building a portfolio, and continuously educating yourself will promote your career growth. Also, embracing industry changes, balancing speed and accuracy, and overcoming challenges will help you thrive in your chosen profession.

Moreover, increasing your earnings by specializing in specific areas and negotiating pay and benefits ensures a fulfilling and financially rewarding career. As you progress, opportunities for leadership and teaching may surface and offer you more avenues for personal and professional development.

Finally, this book aims to motivate you on your journey into the world of medical billing and coding. It is a field with stability, a sense of purpose, and the opportunity to impact healthcare delivery in a positive way. From the author's personal experience, we hope you feel empowered to pursue this exciting career path.

Note that success in medical billing and coding is not just limited to technical proficiency but also requires dedication to accuracy, ethics, and continuous improvement. Face the challenges, be curious, and keep learning. Your journey into the world of medical billing and coding awaits—good luck!

GET YOUR FREE BONUSES

Dear Reader,

First and foremost, thank you for purchasing my book! Your support means the world to me, and I hope you find the information within valuable and helpful in your journey.

As a token of my appreciation, I have included some exclusive gifts that will greatly benefit you in your career.

Your Bonuses:

- **Audiobook**: The audiobook version of this book is ideal for busy people. Listen while commuting, during breaks, or at home to reinforce your knowledge and confidence to pass the certification exam.

- **Pharmacology Comprehensive E-Book.** Expand your knowledge of pharmaceuticals and their interactions, gaining a deeper understanding of the medications and treatments used in healthcare.

- **Medical Prefixes and Suffixes E-Book.** Explore the foundation of medical terminology, unraveling the meanings behind prefixes and suffixes commonly encountered in medical language.

- **Glossary of Terms:** Enjoy a comprehensive Glossary of Terms e-book, ensuring no term or definition is left unexplored. This valuable resource serves as a quick reference guide, facilitating your study and comprehension of medical terminology.

- **100 Digital and Printable Flashcards**: These digital and printable flashcards are an excellent tool to help you study and retain crucial information. They are designed to reinforce your knowledge, boost your confidence, and make learning enjoyable and convenient, whether you're on the go or at home. To use the flashcards, I included a "README File" with the instructions.

I kindly ask you to take a moment to leave an honest review or rating of the book; it takes less than 30 seconds. Your feedback not only helps me improve my future work, but it also assists other readers in making informed decisions about their purchases. Please share your thoughts and experiences, as every review counts!

To access these bonuses, simply click on the link if you're using the e-book version or scan the QR code with your phone if you have the physical copy.

CLICK   HERE   FOR   THE   BONUSES

or

Scan this QR Code

Once again, thank you for your support, and I wish you the best of luck in your medical billing and coding career. I believe these bonuses will provide you with the tools and knowledge to excel in this industry.

If you want to leave an honest review or rating, here's the link for direct access; it takes less than 30 seconds:

CLICK   HERE   TO   LEAVE   A   REVIEW

Or, scan this QR Code below:

Happy reading, and enjoy your bonuses!

CONTACT THE AUTHOR

I always strive to make this guide as comprehensive and helpful as possible, but there's always room for improvement. If you have any questions, suggestions, or feedback, I would love to hear from you. Hearing your thoughts helps me understand what works, what doesn't, and what could be made better in future editions.

To make it easier for you to reach out, I have set up a dedicated email address:

✉ epicinkpublishing@gmail.com

Feel free to email me for:

- Clarifications on any topics covered in this book

- Suggestions for additional topics or improvements

- Feedback on your experience with the book

- Any other inquiries you may have

Your input is invaluable. I read every email and will do my best to respond in a timely manner.

Thank you once again for entrusting me with a part of your educational journey. I wish you all the best in your upcoming exam and future endeavors in the electrical field.

Best wishes

CPC Exam Study Guide 2024

Tests | Q&A |Detailed Explanations

The Ultimate Guide to Crush your CPC EXAM

Table of Contents

BONUS CONTENT

Dear reader,

First and foremost, thank you for purchasing my book! Your support means the world to me, and I hope you find the information within valuable and helpful in your journey.

As a token of my appreciation, I have included some exclusive bonuses that will greatly benefit you. My hope is that this nudges you to give an authentic review. Remember, it only takes a brief moment, and it's invaluable for small publishers.

To access these bonuses, simply click on the link if you're using the ebook version, or scan the QR Code with your phone if you have the physical copy.

CLICK   HERE   FOR   THE   BONUSES

or
Scan this QR Code

Once again, thank you for your support, and I wish you the best of luck in your Exam. I believe these bonuses will provide you with the tools and knowledge to excel.

If you want to leave an honest review/ rating, here's the link for direct   access:

CLICK   HERE   TO   LEAVE   A   REVIEW

Or, Scan this QR Code below

Happy reading, and enjoy your bonuses!

Mastering the CPC Exam: Your Comprehensive Guide to Success in Medical Billing and Coding

"Medicine is not only a science; it is also an art. It does not consist of compounding pills and plasters; it deals with the very processes of life, which must be understood before they may be guided." - Paracelsus

The medical field is a dynamic and rewarding industry that plays a vital role in ensuring quality healthcare for individuals around the globe. As a medical billing and coding professional, you can make an impact by ensuring that doctors and hospitals are reimbursed fairly and accurately, while contributing to the overall functioning of healthcare organizations.

Becoming a medical billing and coding professional can seem like a complex journey, with extensive licensing requirements and a vast amount of knowledge to acquire. The Certified Professional Coder (CPC) exam, conducted by the American Academy of Professional Coders (AAPC), is a critical milestone on this path. It validates your proficiency in medical coding and ensures you are well-equipped to navigate the intricacies of the profession.

We understand that embarking on this journey can be both exciting and daunting. That's why we've created this study guide – to provide you with comprehensive support, guidance, and resources to overcome the hurdles you may encounter on your path to becoming a certified professional coder.

Our aim is to make the CPC exam preparation process approachable and even fun. We've crafted this guide with a friendly and accessible tone, allowing you to delve into the world of medical billing and coding with confidence and ease. Whether you are a newcomer to the field or seeking to enhance your existing knowledge, this study guide is designed to empower you to succeed.

In these pages, you'll find a wealth of information tailored specifically to the CPC exam. We've carefully curated the content to cover all aspects of medical coding, including guidelines, regulations, anatomy, and various coding systems. Each chapter is structured to help you grasp the core concepts, providing real-world examples and practice exercises to reinforce your understanding.

Here's an overview of what you can expect from this study guide:

- **Understanding the Fundamentals:** Lay the foundation of your knowledge by exploring the basics of medical billing and coding. We'll discuss the history, importance, and key roles of medical coders, ensuring you have a solid understanding of the profession.

- **Navigating the Licensing Requirements:** The road to becoming a certified professional coder involves fulfilling specific licensing requirements. We'll guide you through this process and help you understand the prerequisites, exam eligibility criteria, and the application process for the CPC exam.

- **Mastering Medical Terminology:** Acquiring a solid grasp of medical terminology is essential for accurate coding. In this section, we'll dive into the language of medicine and help you develop the necessary vocabulary to decipher complex terminology.

- **Cracking the Coding Systems:** Unravel the complexities of coding systems such as ICD-10-CM, CPT®, and HCPCS Level II. We will explore each system in detail and offer some tips, techniques, and practical examples to enhance your coding skills.

- **Anatomy and Physiology Essentials:** A solid understanding of human anatomy and physiology is vital for accurate coding. We will take a comprehensive journey through the body's systems and highlight some key terms you should know.

- **Exam Strategies and Practice:** Prepare for success with effective exam strategies, time management techniques, and practice questions designed to simulate the CPC exam experience. These resources will help strengthen your coding abilities and build confidence in your knowledge.

With this study guide as your companion, you can approach the CPC exam with confidence, knowing that you have all the necessary tools at your disposal to succeed. Remember, your journey in the medical billing and coding field is a continuous learning process, and this guide serves as a stepping stone to a fulfilling career.

Reasons to Become a Medical Billing and Coding Professional

This section will explore the reasons why pursuing a career in medical billing and coding can be both personally fulfilling and professionally rewarding. As the healthcare industry continues to expand and evolve, the demand for skilled professionals in this field is reaching new heights.

Thanks to booming demand, medical billing and coding professions enjoy competitive salaries and flexible work schedules, with limitless potential for growth. In this section, we'll explore the abundant opportunities available to individuals pursuing a career in medical billing and coding. You'll also play a role in a vital field, ensuring people get the health care they need.

Whether you're seeking stability, intellectual stimulation, or a chance to make a difference in patient care, the path of a medical billing and coding professional is an excellent choice.

Below are just a few reasons to start a career in this challenging, rewarding industry:

Essential Role in Healthcare:
Medical billing and coding professionals serve as the bridge between healthcare providers, insurance companies, and patients. They are responsible for translating complex medical documentation, including diagnoses, procedures, and treatments, into universal codes that are used for billing, reimbursement, and data analysis. Without accurate coding, the

financial health of healthcare organizations and the availability of quality care could be compromised.

High Demand and Career Stability:

The demand for skilled medical billing and coding professionals is on the rise and is expected to continue growing in the coming years. As the healthcare industry expands and undergoes changes, the need for accurate and efficient medical coding becomes even more crucial. This demand translates into excellent career stability and job security for individuals pursuing this profession.

Diverse Employment Opportunities:

Along with growth potential, you'll also enjoy a wide range of employment opportunities. Medical billing and coding professionals can work in various healthcare settings, including hospitals, clinics, physician offices, nursing homes, insurance companies, and government agencies. This versatility allows individuals to choose a work environment that aligns with their preferences and career goals.

Competitive Salary and Benefits:

The strong demand for medical billing and coding professionals means professionals with the right skills usually receive competitive salaries. The average salary for medical billing and coding professionals is around $46,500 a year, although you can earn more with the right certifications and degrees. Many employers also offer benefits such as health insurance, retirement plans, paid time off, and opportunities for professional development and advancement.

Work-Life Balance:

Earning high wages doesn't have to come at the expense of your work-life balance. Many positions in this field offer flexible work schedules, including part-time and remote options. This flexibility can be particularly appealing to those seeking a career that accommodates personal commitments, family obligations, or other interests outside of work.

Intellectual Stimulation and Continuous Learning:

The field of medical billing and coding is intellectually stimulating, providing a constant opportunity for learning and professional growth. As new medical procedures, technologies, and coding guidelines emerge, medical billing and coding professionals must stay abreast of the changes. This dynamic nature of the profession keeps individuals engaged and ensures that their skills remain relevant and valuable.

Contributing to Patient Care:

While medical billing and coding professionals may not provide direct patient care, they significantly impact patient outcomes. Accurate coding ensures that healthcare providers receive proper reimbursement for services rendered, enabling them to continue delivering high-quality care. Additionally, coded data is used for research, analysis, and healthcare planning, ultimately improving patient safety, treatment effectiveness, and population health.

Team Collaboration:

Medical billing and coding professionals help foster collaboration and teamwork in the medical profession. They interact with physicians, nurses, insurance professionals, and administrators to ensure accurate documentation, proper coding, and efficient billing processes. This collaborative environment provides opportunities to build professional relationships, enhance communication skills, and contribute to the success of healthcare teams.

Constantly Evolving Field:

The field of medical billing and coding is always evolving, so you'll always have the opportunity to learn more and advance professionally. Coding systems, guidelines, and regulations are updated regularly to reflect advances in medical practices and technology. Staying up-to-date with these changes ensures that medical billing and coding professionals remain at the forefront of their field and that the job never gets stale.

A Pathway to Specialization:

Medical billing and coding professionals have the opportunity to specialize in various areas of healthcare coding. By pursuing additional certifications or advanced training, individuals can specialize in fields such as anesthesia, cardiology, dermatology, oncology, and more. Specialization allows professionals to focus their expertise and potentially opens doors to more advanced career opportunities and higher compensation.

Overview of the CPC Exam: Your Path to Certification in Medical Billing and Coding

If you've set your sights on becoming a certified professional coder (CPC), the journey ahead may seem challenging. While it isn't easy, the barrier of entry is much lower than many other careers that are less exciting and lucrative.

Fortunately, we're here to guide you through the process. In this section, we'll provide you with a comprehensive overview of the CPC exam, along with an overview of what it takes to succeed.

What is the CPC Exam?

The Certified Professional Coder (CPC) exam is a rigorous assessment designed to evaluate a person's knowledge and proficiency in medical coding. Administered by the American Academy of Professional Coders (AAPC), this exam serves as a benchmark for individuals seeking to become certified professional coders. Achieving CPC certification demonstrates your expertise in accurately translating medical documentation into standardized codes for billing, reimbursement, and data analysis.

The CPC exam is a comprehensive test that assesses your understanding of various coding systems, guidelines, regulations, and medical terminology. It challenges your ability to interpret complex medical scenarios and assign the appropriate codes from systems such as ICD-10-CM (International Classification of Diseases, Tenth Revision, Clinical Modification), CPT® (Current Procedural Terminology), and HCPCS Level II (Healthcare Common Procedure Coding System). The exam consists of 150 multiple-choice questions, and candidates have 5 hours and 40 minutes to complete it.

Why Take the CPC Exam?

You may be wondering why you need to take the CPC exam in the first place. The answer lies in the recognition and validation it provides. CPC certification is widely recognized and respected in the healthcare industry. It demonstrates to employers and colleagues that you have the necessary skills and knowledge to excel in medical billing and coding. Holding this certification opens doors to a multitude of opportunities, including better job prospects, career advancement, and higher earning potential.

Additionally, CPC certification enhances your credibility as a professional coder. It signifies your commitment to maintaining industry standards, ethics, and accuracy in your coding practices. Employers often prioritize certified coders when hiring, knowing that they possess the knowledge required to navigate medical coding with precision and expertise.

Understanding the Exam Structure

The CPC exam consists of 150 multiple-choice questions that assess your understanding of coding principles, guidelines, and real-world medical scenarios. While it's true that the exam is split into two sections, the distinction is not about the use of coding manuals. Instead:

- **Section 1:** Contains 100 questions and focuses on Evaluation and Management (E/M) coding. Candidates cannot use any reference materials for this section.

- **Section 2:** Contains 50 questions and covers a wide range of coding topics beyond E/M, including surgery, radiology, laboratory, medicine, and anesthesia. Candidates can use approved coding manuals for this section.

To successfully pass the CPC exam, you need a solid understanding of:

- **Coding Guidelines:** Official rules and conventions for assigning codes.

- **Medical Terminology:** The language used to describe medical conditions and procedures.

- **Anatomy and Physiology:** The structure and function of the human body.

- **Practical Coding Scenarios:** The ability to apply your knowledge to real-world situations.

Let's face it—the CPC exam can be stressful. It's an extremely important test that requires focused preparation and a thorough understanding of the material. But don't let that discourage you! With the right mindset and diligent study habits, you can overcome the challenges and succeed in this exam.

Studying is extremely importance when preparing for the CPC exam. To succeed, you'll need to do much more than memorize codes. You'll also have to become familiar with underlying concepts, understand coding guidelines, and apply critical thinking skills to real-world coding scenarios. Studying helps you build a solid foundation of knowledge, boosts your confidence, and prepares you to tackle the exam with confidence.

If you plan on taking the CPC exam, it's essential to set aside time for studying. In addition to helping you absorb the material, studying also gives you a chance to identify any knowledge gaps so you can focus on areas that require the most practice.

Effective study techniques include creating a structured study plan, utilizing reputable study materials and resources, practicing with coding scenarios, participating in study groups or forums, and taking advantage of practice exams to assess your progress. Remember to pace yourself, take breaks when needed, and stay motivated by envisioning the rewarding career that awaits you.

Getting Ready for the Test

Pursuing a career in medical billing and coding as a certified professional coder offers some incredible benefits. From stability and competitive pay to the opportunity for personal and professional growth, this field has tremendous potential for motivated people. The CPC exam serves as the gateway to unlocking these opportunities, validating your expertise and knowledge in medical coding.

Embarking on this journey and preparing for the CPC exam is a significant step towards a fulfilling and prosperous career. Studying will help you build the mastery of coding principles and the confidence to succeed in the exam and thrive in the field.

In the next chapter, we'll dive into the basics of medical coding. We'll explore the history, importance, and key roles of medical coders, which will provide you with a solid foundation of knowledge. Through engaging explanations, real-world examples, and practice exercises, we will demystify the coding process and help you set yourself on the path to success.

So, let's proceed to the next chapter, where we will embark on this exciting journey into the fundamentals of medical coding.

Chapter 1: The Basics of Medical Billing and Coding

In this chapter, we'll dive into the an overview of medical billing and coding. If you're thinking of taking the CPC exam, this chapter will provide an overview of what medical coders do and the basics of how they do it.

Medical billing and coding professionals are the behind-the-scenes heroes who ensure that healthcare providers receive accurate reimbursement for the services they render. But what exactly do medical coders do? Well, their primary responsibility is to translate medical documentation, such as diagnoses, procedures, and treatments, into standardized codes.

These codes serve as a common language that allows healthcare providers, insurance companies, and government agencies to communicate and process medical information accurately and efficiently. By assigning the appropriate codes to each medical service or procedure, coders ensure that healthcare providers are reimbursed correctly and that patient records are accurate.

The Role of Certified Professional Coders in the Healthcare System

Doctors and healthcare providers interact most with patients, and almost every hospital or clinic has to work with insurance companies and government agencies. Unfortunately, the healthcare field is full of extremely complicated terminology, which can be confusing even for highly trained doctors and insurance adjusters.

This is where medical billing coders come in. By translating these terms for disorders, anatomical structures, and treatments into standardized codes, they make sure everyone is on the same page. These codes serve as a common language that allows healthcare providers, insurance companies, and government agencies to communicate and process medical information accurately and efficiently.

Certified professional coders help ensure that doctors are paid fairly for their services, according to concrete codes instead of medical terminology, which can cause unnecessary confusion. Below are just a few of the organizations a medical billing and coding professional might work for:

Healthcare Facilities:

Medical billing coders are an integral part of hospitals, clinics, and outpatient facilities. In these settings, they review medical records, extract relevant information, and assign appropriate codes to diagnoses, procedures, and treatments. Accurate coding is essential to facilitate timely and accurate reimbursement for the services provided by healthcare providers. By meticulously assigning the correct codes, medical billing coders help healthcare facilities maintain financial stability, enabling them to deliver quality care and invest in cutting-edge technologies and resources.

Physician Practices:

Medical billing coders play a crucial role in physician practices, including family medicine, pediatrics, cardiology, and many others. They ensure that services rendered by physicians are accurately coded and billed for appropriate reimbursement. By understanding the nuances of different medical specialties and coding guidelines, these professionals contribute to the financial viability of physician practices. Their expertise in accurately translating medical documentation into codes helps practices continue to deliver comprehensive care to patients.

Insurance Companies:

Insurance companies also employ medical billing to review and process claims submitted by healthcare providers. Their expertise ensures that claims are accurately coded and comply with coding guidelines and policy requirements. By meticulously examining medical documentation, medical billing coders play a critical role in determining the appropriateness of reimbursement.

Government Agencies:

Government agencies, such as Medicare and Medicaid, rely on medical billing coders to ensure accurate reimbursement and compliance with coding guidelines. These professionals play a vital role in processing claims, reviewing documentation, and applying the appropriate coding standards. Their expertise helps prevent fraudulent activities and supports the provision of quality care to eligible beneficiaries.

Medical Billing Companies:

Medical billing companies provide specialized services to healthcare providers, managing their billing and coding processes. These companies employ skilled medical billing coders who handle coding, billing, claim submission, and follow-up on behalf of healthcare providers. Outsourcing these functions to medical billing companies allows healthcare providers to focus on patient care while relying on medical billing coders to ensure they're reimbursed.

A Day in the Life of a Billing Coder

The average coding professionals' task starts starts with medical documentation, which can come in the form of physician notes, operative reports, and laboratory results. Coders carefully review this documentation to extract key information that needs to be coded, then uses a coding system to assign codes to each piece of medical information.

These coding systems have specific guidelines and rules that coders must follow to ensure accuracy and compliance. The codes assigned capture crucial details such as the patient's diagnosis, the procedures performed, and any accompanying services or supplies used.

The coded information is then entered into the healthcare organization's billing software or electronic health record system. This ensures that accurate claims are generated for insurance companies and healthcare provider are compensated in a timely manner. Coded data also plays a significant role in research, analysis, and healthcare planning, ultimately benefiting patient care and population health.

As you can see, medical billing and coding professionals are the unsung heroes of the healthcare industry. Their attention to detail, knowledge of coding systems, and adherence to guidelines are essential for accurate billing, reimbursement, and data analysis.

Conclusion

Throughout this chapter, we've explored the vital role that medical billing coders play in the healthcare industry. They are the backbone of the revenue cycle management process, diligently translating complex medical documentation into standardized codes.

The importance of medical billing coders cannot be overstated. Their expertise and attention to detail directly impact the financial health of healthcare organizations. Medical billing coders also contribute to the integrity of insurance programs, government healthcare initiatives, and the overall functioning of the healthcare system.

As we continue our journey into the world of medical billing and coding, the next chapter will delve into the basics of anatomical terms that coders must know. Understanding anatomical terminology is crucial for accurate coding, as it forms the foundation for correctly identifying and describing various body systems, organs, and structures. So, get ready to explore the fascinating intricacies of the human body and its terminology, as we equip you with the knowledge you need to excel as a medical billing coder.

By mastering the fundamentals of medical billing and coding, you are laying the groundwork for a fulfilling and rewarding career in the healthcare industry. The expertise you gain will open doors to various employment opportunities and set you on a path towards professional growth and success.

So, let's proceed to the next chapter, where we will dive into the world of anatomical terms and unlock the language of the human body and expand our coding horizons.

Chapter 2: Human Anatomy and its Application in Medical Coding

Welcome to Chapter 2 of our medical coding journey, where we'll explore the essential knowledge of human anatomy that forms the foundation for accurate medical coding. Understanding human anatomy is crucial for interpreting medical documentation and assigning the appropriate codes, ensuring proper documentation, clear communication, and accurate reimbursement.

In this chapter, we'll delve into the major body systems, anatomical planes and positions, body cavities and regions, anatomical structures, and directional references, equipping you with the knowledge to excel as a medical coder.

Introduction to Human Anatomy

Importance of Understanding Human Anatomy in Medical Coding

In the field of medical coding, human anatomy serves as a roadmap that guides us in accurately assigning codes for medical procedures and conditions. A solid grasp of anatomy enables us to decipher complex medical documentation, ensuring that the correct codes are used for each situation. This accuracy is crucial for proper documentation and clear communication between healthcare providers and insurers.

Overview of the Major Body Systems

The human body is a marvel of interconnected systems working harmoniously to sustain life. Familiarizing yourselves with the major body systems provides insight into the functions of each system and their contributions to overall health. These systems include the cardiovascular system, respiratory system, muscular and skeletal systems, nervous system, and endocrine system. Each of these systems has its own terminology that describes structures, disorders, and medical treatments.

Anatomical Planes and Positions

Anatomical planes are imaginary flat surfaces that divide the body into specific sections. These planes serve as reference points for describing the location and orientation of anatomical structures. Understanding these planes and corresponding body positions is essential for accurately assigning medical codes and interpreting medical documentation.

Anatomical Planes:

- **Sagittal Plane:** A vertical plane that divides the body into left and right halves. If the plane passes directly through the midline, it's called the midsagittal or median plane.

- **Coronal (Frontal) Plane:** A vertical plane that divides the body into anterior (front) and posterior (back) sections.

- **Transverse (Axial or Horizontal) Plane:** A horizontal plane that divides the body into superior (upper) and inferior (lower) sections.

Body Positions:

- **Supine Position:** Lying flat on the back with the face upward.

- **Prone Position:** Lying face down on the stomach.

- **Lateral Position:** Lying on the side, either left lateral (left side down) or right lateral (right side down).

- **Trendelenburg Position:** Lying on the back with the head lower than the feet, often used in surgery or for patients in shock.

- **Fowler's Position:** A semi-sitting position with the head of the bed elevated. There are variations like semi-Fowler's (30-degree elevation) and high Fowler's (90-degree elevation).

Human anatomy includes various body cavities that house and protect essential organs and structures. Understanding these cavities and their regions is crucial for accurate anatomical referencing and medical coding.

Main Body Cavities:

- **Dorsal Cavity:** Located towards the back of the body, it is further divided into:

    o **Cranial Cavity:** Encloses the brain.

    o **Spinal (Vertebral) Cavity:** Encloses the spinal cord.

- **Ventral Cavity:** Located towards the front of the body, it is divided by the diaphragm into:

    o **Thoracic Cavity:** Contains the heart and lungs, each enclosed in their respective pleural cavities, as well as the mediastinum, a central compartment housing the trachea, esophagus, and major blood vessels.

    o **Abdominopelvic Cavity:** Further divided into:

        ▪ **Abdominal Cavity:** Contains organs like the stomach, liver, spleen, pancreas, gallbladder, small intestine, and most of the large intestine.

        ▪ **Pelvic Cavity:** Contains the urinary bladder, reproductive organs, and the remaining part of the large intestine (rectum).

Abdominopelvic Quadrants:

The abdominopelvic cavity can be divided into four quadrants by two imaginary lines intersecting at the umbilicus (belly button):

- **Right Upper Quadrant (RUQ):** Liver, gallbladder, right kidney, and parts of the stomach, pancreas, and intestines.

- **Left Upper Quadrant (LUQ):** Stomach, spleen, left kidney, and parts of the pancreas and intestines.

- **Right Lower Quadrant (RLQ):** Appendix, cecum, right ovary (in females), and parts of the intestines.

- **Left Lower Quadrant (LLQ):** Sigmoid colon, left ovary (in females), and parts of the intestines.

Abdominopelvic Regions (Nine-Region Method):

For more precise localization, the abdominopelvic cavity can be further divided into nine regions using four imaginary lines:

- **Right Hypochondriac:** Liver, gallbladder, and right kidney.

- **Epigastric:** Stomach, liver, pancreas, and duodenum.

- **Left Hypochondriac:** Spleen, left kidney, and parts of the stomach and pancreas.

- **Right Lumbar:** Ascending colon, right kidney, and part of the small intestine.

- **Umbilical:** Transverse colon, small intestine, and duodenum.

- **Left Lumbar:** Descending colon, left kidney, and part of the small intestine.

- **Right Iliac (Inguinal):** Cecum, appendix, and right ovary/spermatic cord.

- **Hypogastric (Pubic):** Urinary bladder, uterus (in females), and sigmoid colon.

- **Left Iliac (Inguinal):** Sigmoid colon, left ovary/spermatic cord.

Anatomical Structures and Terminology

Knowledge of the human body's structures and terminology enables us to identify affected areas and assign appropriate codes. Below are a few key systems and structs you should know about if you're planning on becoming a medical billing coding professional:

- **Cells, Tissues, Organs, and Systems:** The human body functions as a complex network of cells, tissues, organs, and systems. Understanding this hierarchy helps in identifying the affected area and assigning appropriate codes.

- **Bones, Joints, and Muscles:** The skeletal system provides the framework of the body, and knowledge of bones, joints, and muscles is essential for coding fractures, joint disorders, and musculoskeletal procedures.

- **Blood Vessels and Circulation:** The circulatory system comprises blood vessels responsible for oxygen and nutrient distribution. Understanding this system is crucial for coding cardiovascular conditions and related procedures.

- **Nerves and Innervation:** The nervous system facilitates communication within the body. Knowledge of nerves and innervation pathways is essential for coding neurologic conditions and procedures.

- **Glands and Hormones:** The endocrine system regulates bodily functions through hormones. Familiarity with glands and their functions aids in coding endocrine disorders and treatments.

Basic Anatomical Terminology and Directional References

Anatomical terminology and directional references help accurately communicate the location and relationships between anatomical structures. Because medical records must be extremely accurate, doctors and health insurance companies use specific terminology to describe directions and sides of the body.

Medical billing professionals should know the following terms:

- **Anterior (Ventral) and Posterior (Dorsal):** Referring to the front and back of the body, respectively.

- **Superior and Inferior:** Describing structures as upper or lower in position.

- **Medial and Lateral:** Indicating structures' proximity to or distance from the midline of the body.

- **Proximal and Distal:** Referring to structures' closeness or distance to a reference point.

- **Superficial and Deep:** Describing structures' location on the body's surface or within the body.

- **Internal and External:** Indicating structures' position within or outside a particular structure.

- **Bilateral and Unilateral:** Denoting structures or conditions affecting both sides or only one side of the body.

- **Ipsilateral and Contralateral:** Describing structures or conditions occurring on the same side or opposite sides of the body.

Conclusion

As you wrap up this chapter, you've successfully navigated through the intricacies of human anatomy. You should also have developed an understanding of the major body systems, anatomical planes and positions, body cavities and regions, anatomical structures, and directional references. Your newfound knowledge serves as a strong foundation for accurate and efficient medical coding.

By mastering human anatomy, you are now equipped to precisely identify and describe anatomical structures, interpret medical documentation, and assign the appropriate codes. Most importantly, this knowledge can serve as the foundation of a challenging career.

The next chapter will unlock the secrets of medical terminology – the language that enables us to communicate with precision and accuracy in the medical coding universe. This language can seem intimidating, but the tips in the next chapter will help you identify even complex terms with confidence.

Chapter 3: Mastering Medical Terminology in Medical Coding

Medical terminology is the language that unlocks the secrets of medical reports and empowers us to accurately assign codes. Understanding medical terms is like learning a new language, which can seem intimidating at first.

In this section, we'll break medical terminology down into easy-to-digest bites. Learning prefixes and roots and how to combine will make you a medical language expert in no time. We'll also explore a variety of terms related to different body systems and disorders to ensure you're equipped to navigate coding in the dynamic world of healthcare.

Introduction to Medical Terminology

Importance of Medical Terminology in Medical Coding

Medical terminology is the glue that holds medical coding together. Understanding medical terms allows us to accurately interpret medical reports, communicate with healthcare providers, and assign the right codes. It's like having a secret codebook that unlocks the mysteries of patient care and billing.

How Medical Terms are Built

Before we dive into the sea of medical terms, let's equip ourselves with the tools to build them. Medical terms are constructed using three key components: prefixes, roots, and suffixes. It's like building a complex puzzle, where each piece brings meaning to the whole.

Below, we'll explore the role of each component and how they work together to form meaningful medical words.

Prefixes

Medical terminology is like a puzzle, with each word constructed from smaller building blocks: prefixes, roots, and suffixes. Understanding these components unlocks the meaning of complex medical terms, aiding in accurate coding and communication.

Prefixes:

Prefixes are word parts added to the beginning of a term to modify its meaning or provide context. For example:

- **Hypo-:** means "under" or "below normal," as in *hypoglycemia* (low blood sugar).

- **Hyper-:** means "excessive" or "above normal," as in *hypertension* (high blood pressure).

- **A- or An-:** means "without" or "absence of," as in *anemia* (lack of red blood cells).

Roots:

Roots are the foundation of medical terms, providing the core meaning related to a body part, organ, or system. Some common examples include:

- **Cardi/o:** refers to the heart, as in *cardiology* (study of the heart) or *cardiomyopathy* (disease of the heart muscle).

- **Derm/o or Dermat/o:** refers to the skin, as in *dermatology* (study of the skin) or *dermatitis* (inflammation of the skin).

- **Gastr/o:** refers to the stomach, as in *gastritis* (inflammation of the stomach lining) or *gastroenterology* (study of the stomach and intestines).

Suffixes:

Suffixes are added to the end of a term to indicate a condition, procedure, or disease process. Some common suffixes include:

- **-itis:** means "inflammation," as in *appendicitis* (inflammation of the appendix).

- **-ectomy:** means "surgical removal," as in *appendectomy* (surgical removal of the appendix).

- **-oma:** means "tumor" or "mass," as in *carcinoma* (cancerous tumor).

- **-algia:** means "pain," as in *neuralgia* (nerve pain).

Building and Deciphering Medical Terms:

By combining prefixes, roots, and suffixes, you can construct and understand complex medical terms. For example:

- **Hyperthyroidism:** "Hyper-" (excessive) + "thyroid" (thyroid gland) + "-ism" (condition) = overactive thyroid gland.

- **Cardiomegaly:** "Cardio" (heart) + "-megaly" (enlargement) = enlarged heart.

- **Dermatologist:** "Dermato" (skin) + "-logist" (specialist) = a doctor specializing in skin conditions.

Terms Related to Body Systems and Disorders

Now that we've equipped ourselves with the tools to build medical terms, let's dive into exploring terms related to specific body systems and disorders. This knowledge is essential for identifying and coding a patient's medical records. Each body system has a unique set of terms and is subject to a different set of diseases and conditions.

Below is an overview of the most important systems in the human body and some of the terms you might encounter in your coding career.

Cardiovascular System

The cardiovascular system transports oxygen and nutrients to every nook and cranny. Let's explore common cardiovascular terms and learn how to accurately code cardiovascular disorders, ensuring efficient and effective healthcare billing.

Common Cardiovascular Terms

- **Angina:** Chest pain due to reduced blood flow to the heart muscle.

- **Arrhythmia:** Irregular heart rhythm.

- **Atherosclerosis:** Build-up of plaque in the arteries, narrowing the blood vessels.

- **Hypertension:** High blood pressure.

194

- **Myocardial Infarction (Heart Attack):** Blockage of blood flow to the heart muscle, causing damage.
- **Pericarditis:** Inflammation of the lining around the heart.

Coding Cardiovascular Disorders

Cardiovascular conditions are complex and require precise coding for accurate billing and record-keeping. To pass the CPC exam and work effectively as a medical coder, a thorough understanding of the codes for various heart conditions, vascular disorders, and procedures is crucial.

Each code represents a specific medical condition or treatment within the ICD-10-CM (International Classification of Diseases, Tenth Revision, Clinical Modification) system. For example:

- Atrial fibrillation (AFib) has several potential codes depending on the type and cause:
    - I48.0 for paroxysmal AFib
    - I48.1 for persistent AFib
    - I48.2 for chronic AFib
- Congestive heart failure (CHF) also has multiple codes depending on the type and severity:
    - I50.9 for heart failure, unspecified
    - I50.20 for systolic heart failure, unspecified
    - I50.23 for acute on chronic systolic heart failure

Cardiac procedures are coded using CPT (Current Procedural Terminology) codes. Some examples include:

- Coronary angioplasty (PTCA): 92920 is indeed the correct code for a single artery, but for multiple arteries or branches, other codes like 92921-92924 may be applicable depending on the number of vessels treated.

- Coronary stent placement: 92928 is one of several codes used for stent placement. The specific code depends on the number and type of stents used, as well as any additional procedures performed during the same session.

It's important to note that coding guidelines and specific codes may change over time. Staying up-to-date with the latest information and utilizing official coding resources is essential for accurate coding and compliance.

Respiratory System

The respiratory system brings air into the body, extracts oxygen, and expels carbon dioxide. This complex system is subject to a wide range of disorders and diseases, ranging from infections to disorders in the lungs. Below are a few common terms associated with the respiratory system.

Common Respiratory Terms

- **Bronchitis:** Inflammation of the bronchial tubes.

- **Pneumonia:** Infection in the lungs, often caused by bacteria or viruses.

- **Asthma:** Chronic respiratory condition characterized by airway inflammation and constriction.

- **Chronic Obstructive Pulmonary Disease (COPD):** A group of progressive lung diseases, including chronic bronchitis and emphysema.

- **Respiratory Failure:** Inadequate gas exchange in the lungs, leading to low oxygen levels.

- **Pleurisy:** Inflammation of the lining around the lungs.

Coding Respiratory Disorders

Respiratory disorders and their associated treatments are diverse and require specific coding to accurately reflect the patient's condition and the procedures performed. To effectively code for respiratory issues, a thorough understanding of ICD-10-CM and CPT codes is essential.

For instance, asthma, a common respiratory condition, has various codes depending on the type and severity:

- J45.901: Asthma, uncomplicated

- J45.902: Asthma, mild intermittent

- J45.903: Asthma, mild persistent

- J45.904: Asthma, moderate persistent

- J45.905: Asthma, severe persistent

Coding respiratory procedures can be complex due to the variety of techniques and approaches. Some examples include:

- Bronchoscopy: As you mentioned, CPT code 31622 is used for a diagnostic bronchoscopy. However, there are additional codes depending on whether biopsies, washings, or other interventions are performed (e.g., 31625 for bronchoalveolar lavage).

- Chest tube insertion (tube thoracostomy): CPT code 32551 is the correct code for this procedure, as you stated.

Gastrointestinal System

The gastrointestinal system is responsible for digesting and absorbing nutrients for the body's sustenance. As we explore common gastrointestinal terms, you'll become proficient in coding gastrointestinal disorders and procedures.

Common Gastrointestinal Terms

- **Gastritis:** Inflammation of the stomach lining.

- **Gastroenteritis:** Inflammation of the stomach and intestines, often due to infections.

- **Peptic Ulcer Disease:** Sores that develop on the lining of the stomach, small intestine, or esophagus.

- **Inflammatory Bowel Disease (IBD):** Chronic inflammation of the gastrointestinal tract, including Crohn's disease and ulcerative colitis.

- **Gallstones:** Solid particles that form in the gallbladder.

- **Diverticulitis:** Inflammation of small pouches that can form in the walls of the colon.

Coding Gastrointestinal Disorders

Like other parts of the body, gastrointestinal disorders and treatments have their own specific codes. The list below isn't exhaustive, but it does provide a glimpse into this complex category of diseases and medical interventions.

Gastrointestinal (GI) Conditions and ICD-10 Codes

Gastrointestinal (GI) disorders encompass a wide range of conditions affecting the digestive system. Accurate ICD-10 coding is essential for proper diagnosis, treatment, and reimbursement. Here's an updated list of common GI conditions and their associated codes:

Gastritis:

- K29.00: Acute gastritis without bleeding

- K29.01: Acute gastritis with bleeding

- K29.30: Alcoholic gastritis without bleeding

- K29.31: Alcoholic gastritis with bleeding

- K29.50: Chronic gastritis, unspecified, without bleeding

- K29.51: Chronic gastritis, unspecified, with bleeding

- K29.60: Other gastritis without bleeding

- K29.61: Other gastritis with bleeding

- K29.70: Gastritis, unspecified, without bleeding

- K29.71: Gastritis, unspecified, with bleeding

Gastroesophageal Reflux Disease (GERD):

- K21.0: Gastro-esophageal reflux disease with esophagitis
- K21.9: Gastro-esophageal reflux disease without esophagitis

1. www.hcpro.com

www.hcpro.com

Peptic Ulcer Disease (PUD):

- K25.5: Gastric ulcer, acute with hemorrhage
- K25.6: Gastric ulcer, acute with both hemorrhage and perforation
- K25.7: Gastric ulcer, acute without hemorrhage or perforation
- K26.5: Duodenal ulcer, acute with hemorrhage
- K26.6: Duodenal ulcer, acute with both hemorrhage and perforation
- K26.7: Duodenal ulcer, acute without hemorrhage or perforation

Inflammatory Bowel Disease (IBD):

- K50.00: Crohn's disease of small intestine, unspecified, without complications
- K50.10: Crohn's disease of large intestine, unspecified, without complications
- K50.80: Crohn's disease of other site, unspecified, without complications
- K50.90: Crohn's disease, unspecified, without complications

- K51.00: Ulcerative (chronic) pancolitis, without complications

- K51.40: Ulcerative (chronic) proctitis, without complications

- K51.90: Ulcerative colitis, unspecified, without complications

Gastrointestinal Treatments:

⬚ Colonoscopy:

- **CPT Code:** 45378 (Colonoscopy, flexible, proximal to splenic flexure; diagnostic, with or without collection of specimen(s) by brushing or washing, with or without colon decompression (separate procedure)).

⬚ Esophagogastroduodenoscopy (EGD):

- **CPT Code:** 43239 (Esophagogastroduodenoscopy, flexible, transoral; diagnostic, including collection of specimen(s) by brushing or washing, when performed (separate procedure)).

⬚ Gastrostomy Tube Placement:

- **CPT Code:** 43760 has been replaced by CPT codes 43762 and 43763:

    - **43762:** Replacement of gastrostomy tube, percutaneous, includes removal, without imaging or endoscopic guidance; simple.

    - **43763:** Replacement of gastrostomy tube, percutaneous, includes removal, without imaging or endoscopic guidance; complicated (e.g., fractured gastrostomy tube requiring additional work).

⬚ Small Bowel Endoscopy (Single and Double Balloon):

- **CPT Code:** 44360 (Enteroscopy, flexible, proximal to duodenum, diagnostic; with or without collection of specimen(s) by brushing or washing, with or without injection into submucosal tissues, with or without endoscopic ultrasound examination).

⬜ Gastric Bypass Surgery:

- **CPT Code:** 43644 (Laparoscopy, surgical, gastric restrictive procedure; with gastric bypass and Roux-en-Y gastroenterostomy (Roux limb 150 cm or less)).

Musculoskeletal System

The musculoskeletal system is like the sturdy scaffolding of the human body, providing support and enabling movement. This system is prone to a variety of disorders, from traumatic injuries to cancers and other diseases. Below are some of the key terms associated with the musculoskeletal system:

Common Musculoskeletal Terms

- **Osteoarthritis:** Degenerative joint disease, resulting in joint pain and stiffness.

- **Rheumatoid Arthritis:** Autoimmune disease causing joint inflammation and damage.

- **Fracture:** A break in a bone.

- **Sprain:** Injury to a ligament, often due to overstretching.

- **Herniated Disc:** A problem with one of the rubbery cushions (discs) between the individual bones (vertebrae) that stack up to make the spine.

- **Carpal Tunnel Syndrome:** Compression of the median nerve in the wrist, leading to hand pain and numbness.

Coding Musculoskeletal Disorders

Medical coders use a range of codes used by medical billing coders to accurately document and bill for various musculoskeletal conditions and treatments. From common orthopedic disorders to intricate surgical procedures, these codes cover a wide range of conditions and treatments.

Osteoarthritis:

- **M19.90:** Unspecified osteoarthritis, unspecified site

- **M17.9:** Osteoarthritis of knee, unspecified

- **M16.0:** Bilateral primary osteoarthritis of hip

- **M16.1:** Unilateral primary osteoarthritis of hip

- **M16.2:** Bilateral osteoarthritis resulting from hip dysplasia

- **M16.3:** Unilateral osteoarthritis resulting from hip dysplasia

- **M16.4:** Bilateral post-traumatic osteoarthritis of hip

- **M16.5:** Unilateral post-traumatic osteoarthritis of hip

- **M16.6:** Other bilateral secondary osteoarthritis of hip

- **M16.7:** Other unilateral secondary osteoarthritis of hip

- **M16.9:** Osteoarthritis of hip, unspecified (AAPC)

Rheumatoid Arthritis:

- **M05.10:** Rheumatoid arthritis of unspecified site, without organ or systems involvement

- **M06.9:** Rheumatoid arthritis, unspecified

- **M05.9:** Rheumatoid arthritis with rheumatoid factor of unspecified site (Carepatron)

Rotator Cuff Tear:

- **M75.101:** Rotator cuff tear or rupture of right shoulder, not specified as traumatic

- **M75.102:** Rotator cuff tear or rupture of left shoulder, not specified as traumatic

- **M75.121:** Complete rotator cuff tear or rupture of right shoulder, not specified as traumatic

- **M75.122:** Complete rotator cuff tear or rupture of left shoulder, not specified as traumatic (Find-A-Code)

Herniated Disc:

- **M51.36:** Other intervertebral disc displacement, lumbar region

CPT Codes for Musculoskeletal Treatments

Arthroscopy:

- **29822:** Arthroscopy, shoulder, surgical; with partial removal of a bone spur

Joint Injection:

- **20610:** Arthrocentesis, aspiration, and/or injection; major joint or bursa

Fracture Repair:

- **25605:** Open treatment of distal radial fracture (e.g., Colles or Smith type) or epiphyseal separation, includes internal fixation, when performed, includes repair of ulnar styloid, when performed

Total Hip Replacement:

- **27130:** Arthroplasty, acetabular and proximal femoral prosthetic replacement (total hip arthroplasty), with or without autograft or allograft

Spinal Fusion Surgery:

- **22612:** Arthrodesis, posterior interbody technique, including laminectomy and/or discectomy to prepare interspace (other than for decompression), single interspace, lumbar

Nervous System

The nervous system is an intricate communication network that transmits messages between the brain and body. Let's explore common nervous system terms and learn how to accurately code neurologic disorders and procedures.

Common Nervous System Terms

- **Stroke:** A sudden interruption in the blood supply to the brain, leading to brain cell damage.

- **Epilepsy:** A disorder characterized by recurrent seizures.

- **Multiple Sclerosis (MS):** An autoimmune disease that affects the central nervous system, leading to communication problems between the brain and the rest of the body.

- **Peripheral Neuropathy:** Damage to the peripheral nerves, causing weakness, numbness, and pain.

- **Migraine:** A severe headache, often accompanied by sensory disturbances and nausea.

- **Parkinson's Disease:** A progressive disorder of the nervous system that affects movement.

Coding Neurologic Disorders

Neurological disorders are extremely complex and require a long list of detailed codes to differentiate between different disorders and treatments. Below is an overview of some of the codes associated with the nervous system.

Neurological Disorders:

Migraine:

- **G43.909:** Migraine, not elsewhere classified, without intractable migraine, without status migrainosus

204

- **G43.909:** Migraine, unspecified, not intractable, without status migrainosus

- **G43.501:** Migraine, not elsewhere classified, intractable, with status migrainosus

- **G43.509:** Migraine, not elsewhere classified, intractable, without status migrainosus (ICD-10 Coded)

Stroke:

- **I63.9:** Cerebral infarction, unspecified

Epilepsy:

- **G40.901:** Localization-related (focal) (partial) idiopathic epilepsy and epileptic syndromes with seizures of localized onset, not intractable, without status epilepticus

- **G40.909:** Epilepsy, unspecified, not intractable, without status epilepticus (ICD-10 Coded)

- **G40.919:** Epilepsy, unspecified, intractable, without status epilepticus

Multiple Sclerosis (MS):

- **G35:** Multiple sclerosis (ICD-10 Coded)

Neurological Treatments:

CPT Codes for Neurological and Spinal Procedures

Lumbar Puncture:

- **CPT Code 62270:** Spinal puncture, lumbar, diagnostic

- **CPT Code 62272:** Spinal puncture, therapeutic, for drainage of cerebrospinal fluid

- **CPT Code 76942:** Ultrasonic guidance for needle placement (e.g., biopsy, aspiration, injection, localization device), imaging supervision and interpretation

Nerve Conduction Study:

- **CPT Code 95907:** Nerve conduction studies; 1-2 studies

- **CPT Code 95908:** Nerve conduction studies; 3-4 studies

- **CPT Code 95909:** Nerve conduction studies; 5-6 studies

- **CPT Code 95910:** Nerve conduction studies; 7-8 studies

- **CPT Code 95911:** Nerve conduction studies; 9-10 studies

- **CPT Code 95912:** Nerve conduction studies; 11-12 studies

- **CPT Code 95913:** Nerve conduction studies; 13 or more studies

Deep Brain Stimulation (DBS) Surgery:

- **CPT Code 61885:** Insertion or replacement of cranial neurostimulator pulse generator or receiver, direct or inductive coupling; with connection to a single electrode array

- **CPT Code 61886:** Insertion or replacement of cranial neurostimulator pulse generator or receiver, direct or inductive coupling; with connection to two or more electrode arrays (Health tech for the digital age)

Carotid Endarterectomy:

- **CPT Code 35301:** Carotid endarterectomy, with or without patch graft

Lumbar Spinal Fusion:

- **CPT Code 22630:** Arthrodesis, posterior interbody technique, including laminectomy and/or discectomy to prepare interspace (other than for decompression), single interspace, lumbar

- **CPT Code 22632:** Arthrodesis, each additional interspace (List separately in addition to code for primary procedure)

- **CPT Code 22842:** Posterior segmental instrumentation (e.g., pedicle fixation, dual rods with multiple hooks and sublaminar wires); 3 to 6 vertebral segments

- **CPT Code 22843:** Posterior segmental instrumentation (e.g., pedicle fixation, dual rods with multiple hooks and sublaminar wires); 7 to 12 vertebral segments

This list is just a sample of how medical coders work with neurologists and insurance companies to ensure that bills are accurate and processed efficiently. We'll go into more detail and offer additional study guides in later chapters.

Endocrine System

The endocrine system is like a network of hormonal messengers, regulating various bodily functions. As we dive into common endocrine terms, you'll gain the skills to code a variety of endocrine disorders and treatments.

Common Endocrine Terms

- **Diabetes Mellitus:** A group of metabolic disorders characterized by high blood sugar levels.

- **Hypothyroidism:** Underactive thyroid gland, leading to decreased metabolism.

- **Hyperthyroidism:** Overactive thyroid gland, leading to increased metabolism.

- **Addison's Disease:** A condition where the adrenal glands do not produce enough hormones.

- **Cushing's Syndrome:** A condition caused by prolonged exposure to high levels of cortisol (a hormone produced by the adrenal gland).

- **Polycystic Ovary Syndrome (PCOS):** A hormonal disorder common among women of reproductive age, leading to infrequent menstrual periods, excess hair growth, acne, and obesity.

Coding Endocrine Disorders

Endocrine issues can impact almost every system in your body and cause a wide range of disorders and conditions. Medical billing and coding professionals will need to understand a variety of codes. Below are a few terms you should be familiar with.

Endocrine Disorders:

Diabetes Mellitus

- **E11.9:** Type 2 diabetes mellitus without complications
- **E10.9:** Type 1 diabetes mellitus without complications
- **E11.65:** Type 2 diabetes mellitus with hyperglycemia
- **E13.9:** Other specified diabetes mellitus without complications

Thyroid Disorders

- **E03.9:** Hypothyroidism, unspecified
- **E04.9:** Nontoxic goiter, unspecified
- **E07.9:** Disorder of thyroid, unspecified
- **E05.90:** Thyrotoxicosis, unspecified without thyrotoxic crisis or storm

Adrenal Disorders

- **E27.9:** Disorder of adrenal gland, unspecified
- **E25.9:** Adrenogenital disorders, unspecified
- **E27.1:** Primary adrenocortical insufficiency
- **E24.9:** Cushing's syndrome, unspecified

Endocrine Treatments:

Insulin Pump Management

- **CPT Code 95251:** Ambulatory continuous glucose monitoring of interstitial tissue fluid via a subcutaneous sensor for a minimum of 72 hours; interpretation and report

- **CPT Code 95249:** Personal CGM setup and patient training

- **CPT Code 95250:** Professional CGM; sensor placement, hook-up, calibration of monitor, patient training, removal of sensor, and printout of recording

Thyroidectomy

- **CPT Code 60260:** Partial thyroid lobectomy

- **CPT Code 60270:** Thyroid lobectomy; total unilateral

- **CPT Code 60252:** Total thyroidectomy, complete, with limited neck dissection

Hormone Replacement Therapy (HRT)

- **CPT Code 96372:** Therapeutic, prophylactic, or diagnostic injection (specify substance or drug); subcutaneous or intramuscular

Adrenalectomy

- **CPT Code 60540:** Partial adrenalectomy or excision of adrenal tumor

- **CPT Code 60545:** Complete adrenalectomy, unilateral or bilateral

Continuous Glucose Monitoring (CGM)

- **CPT Code 95250:** Ambulatory continuous glucose monitoring of interstitial tissue fluid via a subcutaneous sensor for a minimum of 72 hours; sensor placement, hook-up, calibration of monitor, patient training, removal of sensor, and printout of recording

- **CPT Code 95251:** Ambulatory continuous glucose monitoring of interstitial tissue fluid via a subcutaneous sensor for a minimum of 72 hours; interpretation and report

209

Reproductive System

The reproductive system includes every part of the body that pertains to creating new life. Let's explore common reproductive terms and learn how to accurately code reproductive disorders and procedures, ensuring reproductive health in medical coding.

Common Reproductive Terms

Menorrhagia: Heavy or prolonged menstrual bleeding.

Infertility: The inability to conceive a child.

Prostate Cancer: Cancer of the prostate gland in men.

Uterine Fibroids: Non-cancerous growths of the uterus.

Erectile Dysfunction: The inability to achieve or maintain an erection.

Polycystic Ovaries: Multiple small cysts in the ovaries.

Coding Reproductive Disorders

Reproductive System Disorders:

Polycystic Ovary Syndrome (PCOS):

- ICD-10 Code: E28.2 (Polycystic ovarian syndrome)

Erectile Dysfunction:

- ICD-10 Code: N52.9 (Male erectile dysfunction, unspecified)

c. **Endometriosis:**

- ICD-10 Code: N80.9 (Endometriosis, unspecified)

PCOS Related Codes:

- **ICD-10 Code E28.1:** Androgen excess

- **ICD-10 Code E28.8:** Other ovarian dysfunction

- **ICD-10 Code E28.9:** Ovarian dysfunction, unspecified

Erectile Dysfunction Related Codes:

- **ICD-10 Code N52.0:** Erectile dysfunction due to organic causes

- **ICD-10 Code N52.1:** Erectile dysfunction due to a non-organic cause

Endometriosis Related Codes:

- **ICD-10 Code N80.0:** Endometriosis of uterus

- **ICD-10 Code N80.1:** Endometriosis of ovary

- **ICD-10 Code N80.2:** Endometriosis of fallopian tube

- **ICD-10 Code N80.3:** Endometriosis of pelvic peritoneum

- **ICD-10 Code N80.4:** Endometriosis of rectovaginal septum and vagina

- **ICD-10 Code N80.5:** Endometriosis of intestine

- **ICD-10 Code N80.6:** Endometriosis in cutaneous scar

- **ICD-10 Code N80.8:** Other endometriosis

Reproductive System Treatments

Hysterectomy

- **CPT Code 58150:** Total abdominal hysterectomy (corpus and cervix), with or without removal of tube(s), with or without removal of ovary(s)

- **CPT Code 58180:** Supracervical abdominal hysterectomy (subtotal hysterectomy), with or without removal of tube(s), with or without removal of ovary(s)

- **CPT Code 58260:** Vaginal hysterectomy, for uterus 250 g or less

Vasectomy

- **CPT Code 55250:** Vasectomy, unilateral or bilateral (separate procedure), including postoperative semen examination(s)

In Vitro Fertilization (IVF)

- **CPT Code 58970:** Follicle puncture for oocyte retrieval, any method

- **CPT Code 58974:** Embryo transfer, intrauterine

- **CPT Code 58976:** In vitro fertilization, laboratory and related procedures

Colposcopy

- **CPT Code 57455:** Colposcopy of the entire vagina, with cervix if present, with biopsy(s) of the cervix and endocervical curettage

- **CPT Code 57454:** Colposcopy of the cervix including upper/adjacent vagina; with biopsy(s) of the cervix and endocervical curettage

Breast Biopsy

- **CPT Code 19102:** Biopsy of breast; percutaneous, needle core, not using imaging guidance

- **CPT Code 19103:** Biopsy of breast; percutaneous, automated vacuum assisted or rotating biopsy device, using imaging guidance

- **CPT Code 19081:** Biopsy of breast, with placement of localization device and imaging of the biopsy site, when performed, percutaneous; first lesion, including stereotactic guidance

Urinary System

The urinary system removes waste and helps maintain fluid balance in the body. As we venture into common urinary terms, you'll acquire the skills to code a variety of urinary disorders and procedures.

Common Urinary Terms

- **Urinary Tract Infection (UTI):** An infection in any part of the urinary system.

- **Kidney Stones:** Solid particles that form in the kidneys and can cause severe pain.

- **Chronic Kidney Disease (CKD):** The gradual loss of kidney function over time.

- **Urinary Incontinence:** Involuntary leakage of urine.

- **Renal Failure:** The inability of the kidneys to filter waste and maintain fluid balance.

- **Hematuria:** The presence of blood in the urine.

Coding Urinary Disorders

Urinary System Disorders:

Urinary Tract Infection (UTI)

- **ICD-10 Code N39.0:** Urinary tract infection, site not specified (ICD-10 Coded)

Kidney Stones

- **ICD-10 Code N20.0:** Calculus of kidney

- **ICD-10 Code N20.1:** Calculus of ureter

- **ICD-10 Code N20.2:** Calculus of kidney with calculus of ureter (ICD-10 Coded)

Urinary Incontinence

- **ICD-10 Code N39.3:** Stress incontinence (female)

- **ICD-10 Code N39.41:** Urge incontinence

- **ICD-10 Code N39.42:** Incontinence without sensory awareness

- **ICD-10 Code N39.46:** Mixed incontinence (urge and stress)

Urinary System Treatments:

Kidney Transplant

- **CPT Code 50300:** Renal allotransplantation; implantation of graft

- **CPT Code 50320:** Donor nephrectomy (including cold preservation); open

- **CPT Code 50340:** Donor nephrectomy (including cold preservation); laparoscopic

Cystoscopy

- **CPT Code 52000:** Cystoscopy, diagnostic (separate procedure)

- **CPT Code 52204:** Cystourethroscopy, with biopsy(s) of the bladder

Extracorporeal Shock Wave Lithotripsy (ESWL)

- **CPT Code 50590:** Lithotripsy, extracorporeal shock wave

- **CPT Code 52353:** Cystourethroscopy, with ureteroscopy and/or pyeloscopy; with lithotripsy (ureteral catheterization is included in 50590)

Urethral Sling Procedure

- **CPT Code 57288:** Sling operation for stress incontinence, urethropexy (including transvaginal or transobturator)

- **CPT Code 57287:** Removal or revision of sling for stress incontinence (female)

214

Hemodialysis

- **CPT Code 90935:** Hemodialysis procedure with single physician evaluation

- **CPT Code 90937:** Hemodialysis, repeated evaluation(s) by a physician

Integumentary System

The integumentary system is like a protective shield, guarding against external threats. In this section, we'll explore common integumentary terms and learn how to accurately code integumentary disorders and procedures, ensuring the safeguarding of medical coding.

Common Integumentary Terms

- **Eczema:** Inflammatory skin condition, causing red, itchy, and dry skin.

- **Psoriasis:** Chronic skin condition characterized by red, itchy, and scaly patches.

- **Skin Cancer:** Abnormal growth of skin cells, often due to excessive sun exposure.

- **Dermatitis:** Inflammation of the skin.

- **Pressure Ulcers:** Also known as bedsores, caused by prolonged pressure on the skin.

- **Wound Debridement:** Removal of damaged tissue from a wound to promote healing.

Coding Integumentary Disorders

Integumentary System Disorders:

Dermatitis

- **ICD-10 Code L30.9:** Dermatitis, unspecified

- **ICD-10 Code L30.0:** Nummular dermatitis

- **ICD-10 Code L30.8:** Other specified dermatitis

Psoriasis

- **ICD-10 Code L40.9:** Psoriasis, unspecified

- **ICD-10 Code L40.0:** Plaque psoriasis

- **ICD-10 Code L40.1:** Pustular psoriasis

- **ICD-10 Code L40.3:** Palmoplantar psoriasis

- **ICD-10 Code L40.4:** Guttate psoriasis

- **ICD-10 Code L40.5:** Arthropathic psoriasis

Acne

- **ICD-10 Code L70.9:** Acne, unspecified

- **ICD-10 Code L70.0:** Acne vulgari

Integumentary System Treatments:

Excision of Skin Lesion

- **CPT Code 11400:** Excision, benign lesion including margins, except skin tag (unless listed elsewhere), trunk, arms, or legs; excised diameter 0.5 cm or less

- **CPT Code 11401:** Excision, benign lesion including margins, except skin tag (unless listed elsewhere), trunk, arms, or legs; excised diameter 0.6 to 1.0 cm

- **CPT Code 11646:** Excision, malignant lesion including margins, trunk, arms, or legs; excised diameter 4.1 to 5.0 cm

Skin Biopsy

- **CPT Code 11100:** Biopsy of skin, subcutaneous tissue and/or mucous membrane (including simple closure), unless otherwise listed; single lesion

- **CPT Code 11101:** Biopsy of skin, subcutaneous tissue and/or mucous membrane (including simple closure), unless otherwise listed; each additional lesion

- **CPT Code 11102:** Tangential biopsy of skin; single lesion

- **CPT Code 11103:** Tangential biopsy of skin; each separate/additional lesion

- **CPT Code 11104:** Punch biopsy of skin; single lesion

- **CPT Code 11105:** Punch biopsy of skin; each separate/additional lesion

- **CPT Code 11106:** Incisional biopsy of skin; single lesion

- **CPT Code 11107:** Incisional biopsy of skin; each separate/additional lesion

Mohs Micrographic Surgery

- **CPT Code 17311:** Mohs micrographic technique, including removal of all gross tumor, surgical excision of tissue specimens, mapping, color coding of specimens, microscopic examination of specimens by the surgeon, and histopathologic preparation including routine stains, head, neck, hands, feet, genitalia; first stage

- **CPT Code 17312:** Mohs micrographic technique, each additional stage after the first, head, neck, hands, feet, genitalia

- **CPT Code 17313:** Mohs micrographic technique, trunk, arms, legs; first stage

- **CPT Code 17314:** Mohs micrographic technique, each additional stage after the first, trunk, arms, legs

Skin Grafting

- **CPT Code 15100:** Split-thickness autograft, face, scalp, eyelids, mouth, neck, ears, orbits, genitalia, hands, feet, and/or multiple digits, first 100 sq cm or less, or 1% of body area of infants and children

- **CPT Code 15101:** Split-thickness autograft, face, scalp, eyelids, mouth, neck, ears, orbits, genitalia, hands, feet, and/or multiple digits, each additional 100 sq cm or each additional 1% of body area of infants and children (List separately in addition to code for primary procedure)

Conclusion

In this chapter, we've explored how medical terms are built, dissected complex words, and learned how these linguistic building blocks play a crucial role in our daily coding tasks.

By understanding prefixes, root words, and suffixes, we've unlocked the secret to deciphering the meaning of countless medical terms. From gastroenterology to neurosurgery, we now possess the tools to break down these terms and comprehend their significance. It's like becoming fluent in a unique medical language that enables us to communicate effectively with healthcare professionals, insurers, and other members of the medical community.

We've also explored the various body systems, from the cardiovascular to the respiratory, and discovered how each term relates to medical coding. As medical billing coders, this knowledge empowers us to accurately assign codes to different conditions and treatments.

As we continue our journey in the ever-evolving field of medical billing and coding, let's remember that our grasp of medical terminology is the backbone of our profession. With each code we assign and each term we learn, we contribute to a healthier, well-connected world of healthcare.

Now, get ready to embark on the next chapter, where we'll explore the different coding systems that form the foundation of medical billing and coding. From ICD-10 to CPT, we'll uncover the intricacies of these systems and learn how they contribute to our coding endeavors.

Chapter 5: An Introduction to Medical Coding Systems

In this chapter, we'll cover the two fundamental coding systems that form the backbone of our profession: HCPCS (Healthcare Common Procedure Coding System) and ICD-10 (International Classification of Diseases, 10th Revision). These coding systems are used throughout the healthcare profession to provide seamless communication among healthcare professionals, insurers, and other stakeholders.

Understanding HCPCS:

HCPCS, pronounced "hick-picks," is a coding system developed by the Centers for Medicare and Medicaid Services (CMS) to standardize the reporting of healthcare procedures, services, and supplies. It consists of two levels: Level I and Level II.

Level I HCPCS Codes (CPT Codes):

Level I HCPCS codes, also known as CPT codes (Current Procedural Terminology), are maintained and copyrighted by the American Medical Association (AMA). CPT codes primarily represent medical procedures and services provided by healthcare professionals, such as physicians and surgeons.

Examples of Level I HCPCS (CPT) Codes:

Office Visit

- **CPT Code 99213:** This code is used for an office visit with an established patient. It describes a low level of complexity in the evaluation and management of the patient's condition and typically involves 20-29 minutes of total time spent on the encounter. Recent updates for 2024 specify that the code now reflects total time spent on the date of the encounter rather than a time range

Knee Arthroscopy

- **CPT Code 29881:** This code describes knee arthroscopy with meniscectomy (medial or lateral, including any meniscal shaving). It is used for the examination and treatment of the knee joint using an arthroscope

Additional Related Codes

Office Visits:

- **CPT Code 99212:** An office or other outpatient visit to evaluate and manage an established patient requires 10-19 minutes of total time.

- **CPT Code 99214:** An office or other outpatient visit to evaluate and manage an established patient requires 30-39 minutes of total time.

- **CPT Code 99215:** Office or other outpatient visit for the evaluation and management of an established patient, requiring 40-54 minutes of total time

Knee Arthroscopy:

- **CPT Code 29880:** Arthroscopy, knee, surgical; with meniscectomy (medial AND lateral, including any meniscal shaving)

- **CPT Code 29882:** Arthroscopy, knee, surgical; with meniscus repair (medial or lateral)

Level II HCPCS Codes:

Level II HCPCS codes are used for reporting medical supplies, durable medical equipment (DME), and non-physician services, among other items. They are alphanumeric and are commonly used for items not covered by CPT codes.

Examples of Level II HCPCS Codes:

Wheelchair

- **HCPCS Code E0955:** This code is used for billing a manual wheelchair back cushion that is adjustable. It is intended to enhance a patient's mobility and comfort.

Nebulizer

- **HCPCS Code E0570:** This code is used for a nebulizer with a compressor, which is a device that delivers medication in mist form for treating respiratory conditions.

Additional Related Codes:

Wheelchair:

- **E1232:** Manual wheelchair, pediatric size, adjustable

- **E1233:** Manual wheelchair, pediatric size, tilt-in-space

Nebulizer:

- **E0572:** Aerosol compressor, adjustable pressure, light duty for intermittent use

- **E0575:** Nebulizer, ultrasonic, large volume

When to Use HCPCS:

HCPCS is widely used in the United States, particularly in Medicare and Medicaid billing. Medical billing coders must be familiar with HCPCS codes, as they are critical for accurately documenting the specific services and supplies provided to patients. HCPCS codes are particularly valuable when billing for DME, laboratory tests, injections, and other non-physician services.

Navigating ICD-10 Coding System:

The ICD-10 coding system, maintained by the World Health Organization (WHO), is used to classify and code diseases, injuries, and other health conditions. It is an integral part of healthcare documentation, helping to track and analyze health trends, improve patient care, and facilitate accurate billing and reimbursement.

ICD-10 codes consist of alphanumeric characters, typically in the format of a letter followed by two or more numbers. The codes are organized into chapters, blocks, categories, and subcategories, creating a hierarchical structure that allows for a detailed and systematic classification of health conditions.

First Character (Letter): The first character in the ICD-10 code represents the chapter or category. There are 21 chapters in ICD-10, each covering specific body systems or disease groups. For example, Chapter I (A00-B99) covers certain infectious and parasitic diseases, while Chapter IX (E00-E89) is dedicated to endocrine, nutritional, and metabolic diseases.

Second Character (Number): The second character provides further specificity within the chapter or category. It narrows down the classification to a specific block of conditions. For instance, in Chapter IX, the range E10-E14 represents diabetes mellitus, while the range E15-E16 covers other disorders of glucose regulation.

Third and Fourth Characters (Numbers): These characters offer additional detail within the block or category. They specify the particular condition or group of conditions. Continuing with the example from Chapter IX, the code E11.0 represents type 2 diabetes mellitus with ketoacidosis, and E11.9 is used when the type of diabetes is unspecified.

ICD-10 Examples:

Let's explore some examples of ICD-10 codes to gain a better understanding of how this system works:

J45.20 - Unspecified asthma, uncomplicated:

- In this code, "J" represents the chapter for diseases of the respiratory system, specifically asthma.

- The "45" narrows it down to the category for asthma and status asthmaticus.

- "20" specifies that the asthma is unspecified and uncomplicated.

S72.10 - Unspecified fracture of the femur:

- "S" denotes the chapter for injuries to the hip and thigh.

- "72" represents the category for fractures of the femur.

- "10" specifies that the fracture is unspecified.

C50.912 - Malignant neoplasm of upper-outer quadrant of right female breast:

- "C" indicates the chapter for neoplasms or tumors.

- "50" narrows it down to the category for malignant neoplasm of the breast.

- "912" specifies the specific location within the breast, in this case, the upper-outer quadrant of the right female breast.

When to Use ICD-10:

ICD-10 codes are used to report a patient's diagnosis or condition, supporting the medical necessity of services provided. These codes are integral to medical billing, as they influence the reimbursement process and help insurers determine the appropriateness of payment for specific treatments. ICD-10 codes are also crucial for epidemiological research, healthcare statistics, and public health monitoring.

In summary, both HCPCS and ICD-10 coding systems are indispensable in the field of medical billing and coding. While HCPCS codes focus on procedures, supplies, and non-physician services, ICD-10 codes delve into the realm of diagnoses and health conditions. Understanding the nuances of these coding systems empowers medical billing coders to accurately document and communicate crucial healthcare information, facilitating comprehensive and efficient patient care.

Conclusion

With our grasp of HCPCS and ICD-10 coding, we have the power to unlock the mysteries of medical billing, one code at a time. As we continue our journey, let's embrace the knowledge we've gained and prepare to explore even more coding systems and intricacies in the fascinating world of medical billing and coding.

These systems include a great deal of information, but with the right resources and dedication, you can pass the CPC exam with flying colors. In the next section, we'll cover some effective study tips that will help ensure you're prepared for the exam.

Chapter 6: Studying for the CPC Exam

The CPC exam is an intensive, exhaustive test, which can make it seem like a roadblock to an exciting career. While preparing for the CPC exam may seem daunting, being organized and using proven study methods will maximize your chances of success. This chapter will equip you with the smartest study strategies and effective memorization techniques to ace the exam with confidence.

Smart Study Strategies for CPC Exam Prep

Before diving into your study journey, it's important to understand the format of the CPC exam. The exam consists of multiple-choice questions (MCQs), and you'll have a specific amount of time to complete it. Understanding the content areas and how questions are distributed will help you allocate study time wisely.

Below are a few things you should know about the format of the test:

1. **Multiple Choice Questions (MCQs):** MCQs require you to choose the best answer from multiple options. Pay close attention to keyword nuances in the questions and answers to identify the most accurate response.

2. **Time Allocation:** With a limited time for the exam, allocate your time wisely for each section. Don't spend too much time on a single question, and ensure you have time for review at the end.

3. **Content Areas:** The CPC exam covers various coding topics, including evaluation and management (E/M), surgery, medicine, and more. Be aware of the percentage of questions devoted to each area to focus your study efforts effectively.

Creating a Study Plan

A well-structured study plan is your secret weapon for CPC exam success. Below signing up for a test and opening the books, follow the steps below to create a personalized study plan:

1. **Assess Your Current Knowledge:** Before setting study goals, assess your current knowledge of medical coding concepts. Identify your strengths and weaknesses, as this will help you prioritize your focus areas. Take a practice CPC exam or use study resources with self-assessment quizzes to gauge your understanding.

2. **Be Specific and Time-Bound:** Set specific study goals with clear targets and deadlines. Instead of a vague goal like "I want to study CPT codes," specify which CPT sections or chapters you will cover and by what date. Being time-bound adds a sense of urgency and helps you stay on track.

3. **Prioritize Study Goals:** Identify high-priority study goals based on the content areas you find most challenging or that carry more weight in the CPC exam. Focus on areas that contribute significantly to the overall exam score and those that align with your career goals.

4. **Be Realistic:** Set achievable study goals that align with your schedule and commitments. Consider factors like work, family, and other responsibilities when determining how much time you can dedicate to studying each day or week. Avoid overloading yourself with unrealistic expectations.

5. **Seek Support:** Don't hesitate to seek support from mentors, study buddies, or online forums. Engaging with others can provide motivation, insights, and different study perspectives. Additionally, consider joining a CPC study group or enrolling in a review course to gain expert guidance and enhance your study experience.

6. **Utilize Study Resources:** Explore various study resources such as CPC review courses, coding books, online practice tests, and coding forums. A combination of resources will enrich your learning experience.

Practicing with Mock Exams

Practice makes perfect! Fortunately, a variety of online resources and books offer practice exams, many of which are based on actual CPC tests. There are several practice questions in later chapters, but you can also take advantage of other resources to practice and gauge your progress. Here's how to use these valuable resources:

1. **Take Online Practice Tests:** Find reputable online platforms that offer CPC practice exams. These simulate the real exam experience, allowing you to familiarize yourself with the test format. While the questions on these practice tests may not appear on the actual exam, they're usually taken from past versions of the rest.

2. **Review Your Results:** After each practice exam, review your answers and identify areas where you need improvement. When looking at your results, see whether there are any similarities between the questions you missed. This can help you focus your studies and maximize the results of your efforts.

3. **Identify Weak Areas:** Practice tests are instrumental for identifying weak areas. You might score lower on certain topics, or tend to miss questions around certain coding areas. Once you understand your own weak areas, devote more study time to these points and create achievable goals.

Focusing Your Study Sessions:

Coding concepts can be complex, which can be extremely overwhelming, especially when you're trying to absorb walls of information at once. Carefully focusing your study sessions will make this information more manageable and maximize your chances for success. Below are a few tips for making your study sessions more focused:

1. **Break Down Complex Topics:** When faced with complicated topics, break them down into smaller, more manageable parts. In each session, concentrate on a single anatomical system or section of codes. Understanding each component will make tackling the bigger picture easier.

2. **Prioritize Difficult Concepts:** When studying, you might be tempted to focus on areas that seem easier. However, putting off difficult material will slow down your progress. Instead, identify concepts that challenge you the most and prioritize studying them. Give these areas extra time and attention to build a strong foundation.

3. **Utilize Study Groups:** Studying on your own can be difficult, especially if you have trouble staying motivated or focused. Joining study groups with peers can be incredibly beneficial. This will give you a chance to share tips and advice, discuss difficult concepts, and

stay focused on your studies. Having a peer group will also give you someone to help you understand more difficult concepts.

General Techniques for Memorizing Concepts

Succeeding at the CPC exam requires memorizing a great deal of detailed information. This can seem like a Herculean task, but there are simple strategies that can help you commit entire lists of data to memory. Below are a few tips and strategies for boosting your memory retention:

Utilize Mnemonics

Mnemonics are fun and powerful memory aids that can help you remember complex information. They might involve creating acronyms or rhymes that refer to other information. Here are a few fun mnemonic devices to try:

1. **Create Acronyms:** Develop acronyms to remember lists or sequences of information. For example, "RICE" stands for Rest, Ice, Compression, and Elevation - a mnemonic used to remember treatment steps for sprains. Acronyms can help you instantly recall even the most complex information.

2. **Develop Visual Associations:** Associate medical terms or codes with vivid mental images to help them stick in your memory. For instance, you may need to remember the term "rhinorrhea," which means a runny nose. Visualize a rhino (rhino) with a faucet attached to its nose (rhinorrhea) dripping water like a runny nose.

3. **Come Up with Rhymes and Phrases:** Craft rhymes or memorable phrases that incorporate medical terms or coding rules. This can make recalling information more enjoyable and effective. For instance, here's a little poem that helps you remember the steps of coding neoplasm cases in ICD-10:

Neoplasm coding can be a blast

First, check if it's benign or vast.

If it's malignant and you're unsure,

Look for the site and stage to be sure.

Behavior codes come next in line,

Primary or secondary, that's the sign.

Then top it off with the histology,

ICD-10 coding, a breeze, you'll see!

Repetition and Review

Repetition is a powerful tool for memory retention. The more you see, hear, and recall a piece of information, the easier it will be to remember later. Below are a few tips for incorporating repetition into your study routine:

1. **Flashcards and Note-taking:** Create flashcards with coding concepts and review them regularly. If you find yourself struggling to remember specific information, add that information to your list of flash cards. Taking concise notes during your study sessions will also reinforce your learning.

2. **Regular Review Schedule:** Set up a review schedule to revisit coding topics at regular intervals. Spaced repetition - reviewing information at increasing intervals - helps solidify knowledge in the long term. Regularly reviewing your material will help you avoid forgetting information you already committed to memory.

3. **Spaced Repetition Technique:** Instead of cramming all the material in one session, spaced repetition helps reinforce memory by spacing out the review sessions over time. Initially, you review the material

231

frequently, and as you demonstrate better retention, the intervals between reviews are extended.

Applying Concepts to Real-life Scenarios

Applying concepts to real-life scenarios is a powerful way to solidify your understanding of medical coding principles. By practicing coding in context, you'll develop the skills needed to handle complex cases in the real world. Here's how you can apply concepts to various scenarios:

1. **Practical Application:** Take real patient case studies and apply your coding knowledge to assign the appropriate diagnosis and procedure codes. For instance, imagine a patient with a history of diabetes presenting with a foot ulcer and hypertension. Practice coding this scenario by selecting the correct ICD-10 codes for diabetes, foot ulcer, and hypertension, along with any relevant CPT codes for treatment.

2. **Case Studies:** Engage in case studies that mirror real medical scenarios encountered in healthcare settings. For example, work through a case study involving a patient with chest pain, shortness of breath, and a history of heart disease. Code the appropriate E/M visit level, cardiac diagnostic tests, and any subsequent procedures or treatments.

3. **Simulated Coding Exercises:** Participate in simulated coding exercises using coding software or platforms. These exercises mimic real-world coding challenges and often include a variety of coding scenarios. Practice coding scenarios for different specialties, such as orthopedics, dermatology, or cardiology, to gain exposure to diverse medical cases.

4. **Provider Documentation Review:** Review actual medical documentation from healthcare providers, such as progress notes, operative reports, and discharge summaries. Analyze the documentation to extract the necessary information for coding. Familiarize yourself with common abbreviations and medical terms to accurately translate the clinical language into coding language.

Teaching Others

Teaching concepts to others is a powerful way to reinforce your own understanding:

1. **Explaining Concepts to Peers:** Teach coding concepts to study buddies or classmates. The act of teaching requires you to organize your knowledge and clarify your understanding.

2. **Participating in Study Groups:** Joining study groups where participants teach each other can provide a supportive learning environment and fresh insights.

3. **Peer-to-Peer Tutoring:** Offer to tutor peers in coding topics you excel in. Explaining concepts to others solidifies your understanding and fosters a sense of accomplishment.

Strategies for Taking Multiple Choice Tests

Taking multiple-choice tests, such as the CPC exam, requires a specific approach to ensure success. Whether you're sitting for the exam or taking practice tests, here are some valuable strategies to enhance your performance and confidence when tackling multiple-choice questions:

Read Carefully and Analyze: Take your time to read each question thoroughly and understand what it is asking. Pay attention to keywords and qualifiers like "not," "always," or "except," as they can significantly impact the correct answer.

233

Identify the main issue or scenario presented in the question. Often, multiple-choice questions are designed to test your ability to apply concepts to real-life situations.

Eliminate Distractors: Before selecting your answer, eliminate any clearly incorrect options. By narrowing down the choices, you increase the likelihood of selecting the correct answer. Focus on eliminating options that are irrelevant, contain inaccurate information, or contradict the question's context.

Use the Process of Elimination: When you are unsure of the correct answer, use the process of elimination to narrow down your choices. Eliminate any options that are unlikely to be correct, and then make an educated guess among the remaining choices.

Remember that you have a 25% chance of guessing correctly on a four-option multiple-choice question, but you can improve those odds by eliminating incorrect options.

Watch for Modifiers and Exceptions: Pay attention to modifiers such as "usually," "sometimes," or "rarely." These words indicate exceptions to general rules, so be cautious when selecting your answer.

Look for clues in the question that suggest specific guidelines or exceptions, as they can help you arrive at the correct answer.

Beware of Unnecessary Details: In some cases, questions may contain irrelevant information designed to distract you. Focus on the essential elements of the question and avoid getting sidetracked by unnecessary details.

Answer Every Question: In most multiple-choice tests, there is no penalty for guessing. If you are unsure of the correct answer, make an educated guess rather than leaving the question unanswered.

Use the process of elimination and your best judgment to select the most plausible option.

Trust Your Initial Instinct: Often, your initial gut feeling about an answer is correct. Avoid second-guessing yourself, as overthinking can lead to unnecessary mistakes.

Unless you have a solid reason to change your answer, trust your first choice.

Manage Your Time Wisely: Be mindful of the time allocated for the exam. If you encounter a challenging question, flag it and move on to other questions. Return to the flagged questions if you have time left after completing the rest of the exam.

Pace yourself throughout the exam to ensure that you have sufficient time to review your answers if possible.

Stay Calm and Composed: Test anxiety can negatively impact your performance. Take deep breaths and maintain a positive attitude throughout the exam.

If you encounter a challenging question, take a moment to calm yourself before proceeding.

Review Your Answers: If time permits, review your answers before submitting the exam. Look for any errors or overlooked details.

Resist the temptation to change answers unless you are certain of an error.

By incorporating these strategies into your test-taking approach, you'll be better equipped to handle the challenges of multiple-choice exams like the CPC. Practice applying these techniques during mock exams and sample questions to refine your skills and increase your chances of success.

Conclusion

Congratulations on completing this chapter and learning valuable study tips and strategies for the CPC exam! Remember, success in the CPC exam comes from a combination of dedicated preparation, thoughtful study techniques, and a positive mindset. It's normal to feel nervous or overwhelmed, but the techniques in this chapter can help you succeed.

Throughout this chapter, we've explored smart study strategies, memorization techniques, and ways to apply your coding knowledge to real-life scenarios. You've taken significant steps toward CPC exam success by creating a well-structured study plan, practicing with mock exams, and mastering difficult topics.

As you continue your journey, embrace a growth mindset and approach each study session with enthusiasm and determination. Keep in mind that everyone's learning pace is unique, so trust in your progress and celebrate the small victories along the way.

The next chapter will provide you with invaluable practice tests to sharpen your skills and build your confidence further. Practice tests not only gauge your knowledge but also simulate the actual CPC exam experience. You'll get a feel for the exam format, timing, and types of questions you'll encounter, enabling you to fine-tune your approach and optimize your performance.

Don't forget to take breaks when needed and take care of yourself during this preparation period. Rest and relaxation are essential for maintaining focus and mental clarity. You've put in the effort, and it's time to trust in your abilities.

Remember, the CPC exam is an opportunity to showcase your knowledge and skills as a medical billing and coding professional. Approach it with confidence, knowing that you've put in the work to be well-prepared.

Stay determined, stay focused, and remember that you're capable of achieving your goals. The CPC certification is within your reach, and soon, you'll be proudly holding that certificate in your hands!

The Power of Practice Tests

Taking practice tests is an indispensable tool for CPC exam preparation. Practice tests offer numerous benefits that can significantly enhance your performance and confidence on the actual exam day. Here are some compelling reasons why incorporating practice tests into your study routine is essential:

1. **Assessment of Knowledge**: Practice tests provide a way to assess your knowledge and identify areas where you may need additional review. By simulating the exam environment, they help you gauge your level of readiness.

2. **Familiarization with Exam Format**: Practice tests mimic the format of the CPC exam, giving you a sense of what to expect on the big day. Familiarity with the exam structure can reduce test anxiety and help you feel more comfortable during the actual exam.

3. **Time Management Skills**: The CPC exam has a time limit, and practicing with time constraints can improve your ability to manage time efficiently. This skill is crucial for completing the exam within the allotted time.

4. **Real-Life Application of Knowledge**: Practice tests present you with real-life coding scenarios, helping you apply your coding knowledge to practical situations. This reinforces your understanding and prepares you for handling coding challenges in the healthcare setting.

5. **Identifying Weak Areas**: Through practice tests, you can identify areas of weakness and concentrate on reinforcing those concepts during your study sessions. This targeted approach allows for focused improvement.

6. **Building Confidence**: As you consistently perform well on practice tests, your confidence will grow. Confidence is a key factor in reducing test anxiety and performing at your best.

The Features of Practice Tests

1. **Multiple Choice Questions (MCQs)**: Like the CPC exam, practice tests typically consist of multiple-choice questions. These questions present you with several options, and you must select the correct answer.

2. **Varied Content Areas**: Practice tests cover various content areas, including medical terminology, anatomy and physiology, ICD-10 and CPT coding guidelines, and specific coding scenarios.

3. **Timed Sessions**: Some practice tests are timed to simulate the actual exam conditions. Practicing with a time limit will help you gauge your pace and improve time management.

4. **Diagnostic Reports**: Some practice tests offer diagnostic reports after completion, which provide feedback on your performance and highlight areas that need improvement.

5. **Instant Feedback**: Many practice tests provide immediate feedback on each question, indicating whether your answer is correct or incorrect. This instant feedback helps reinforce learning.

:

1. **Which ICD-10-CM code is used for essential (primary) hypertension?**
   A. E11
   B. I10
   C. J45
   D. M19

2. **What is the ICD-10-CM code for Type 2 diabetes mellitus without complications?**
   A. E11.9
   B. E10.9
   C. E11.65
   D. E08.9

3. **Which code is used for a patient with acute bronchitis due to Mycoplasma pneumoniae?**
   A. J20.0
   B. J18.9
   C. J44.9
   D. J45.909

4. **The ICD-10-CM code for major depressive disorder, recurrent, severe without psychotic features is:**
   A. F32.9
   B. F33.2
   C. F31.9
   D. F33.3

5. **What is the correct ICD-10-CM code for chronic obstructive pulmonary disease (COPD)?**
   A. J44.9
   B. J43.0
   C. J45.909
   D. J18.0

6. **Which ICD-10-CM code is used for Alzheimer's disease, unspecified?**
   A. G30.9

B. G30.1

C. F02.80

D. F03.90

7. **What ICD-10-CM code represents uncomplicated acute cystitis?**

    A. N30.00

    B. N39.0

    C. N10

    D. N30.01

8. **Which code is used for a first-degree burn on the right forearm?**

    A. T22.111A

    B. T21.31XA

    C. T20.10XA

    D. T22.111D

9. **What ICD-10-CM code would be used for a patient with severe persistent asthma with status asthmaticus?**

    A. J45.50

    B. J45.21

    C. J45.22

    D. J45.902

10. **Which code represents an encounter for screening mammogram for breast cancer?**

    A. Z12.31

    B. Z12.39

    C. Z12.11

    D. Z13.9

11. **The ICD-10-CM code for a patient diagnosed with Parkinson's disease is:**

    A. G20

    B. G30.0

    C. G35

    D. F03.90

12. **What is the ICD-10-CM code for hyperlipidemia, unspecified?**

    A. E78.5

    B. E78.0

C. E78.2
D. E10.9

13. Which ICD-10-CM code is assigned for gastroesophageal reflux disease (GERD) without esophagitis?

A. K21.0
B. K21.9
C. K20.8
D. K25.9

14. What is the correct code for a patient with a urinary tract infection (UTI), site not specified?

A. N39.0
B. N30.91
C. N10
D. R31.9

15. The ICD-10-CM code for rheumatoid arthritis, unspecified, is:

A. M05.9
B. M06.9
C. M17.9
D. M19.90

16. Which code is used for a diagnosis of obesity, unspecified?

A. E66.9
B. E66.01
C. E66.1
D. E66.8

17. What ICD-10-CM code is used for iron deficiency anemia, unspecified?

A. D50.9
B. D52.9
C. D51.3
D. D53.1

18. Which ICD-10-CM code applies to migraine without aura, not intractable, without status migrainosus?

A. G43.909
B. G43.9090

C. G43.10
D. G43.919

19. What is the ICD-10-CM code for hypertension with heart failure?

A. I10

B. I50.9

C. I11.0

D. I13.10

20. Which ICD-10-CM code is used for an encounter for immunization?

A. Z23

B. Z00.00

C. Z02.89

D. Z21

21. What is the ICD-10-CM code for a fracture of the right femur, initial encounter for closed fracture?

A. S72.001A

B. S72.021A

C. S72.10XA

D. S72.141A

22. Which ICD-10-CM code would you use for acute viral hepatitis B without delta-agent and without hepatic coma?

A. B18.1

B. B19.20

C. B16.9

D. B15.9

23. What is the ICD-10-CM code for anxiety disorder, unspecified?

A. F41.1

B. F41.9

C. F43.21

D. F42.0

24. Which ICD-10-CM code is assigned for chronic kidney disease, stage 3?

A. N18.1

B. N18.3

C. N18.5

D. N18.9

25. **What code is used for a patient presenting with acute pancreatitis?**
    A. K85.9
    B. K86.1
    C. K87.0
    D. K80.0

26. **The ICD-10-CM code for uncomplicated influenza due to unidentified influenza virus is:**
    A. J11.1
    B. J10.1
    C. J09.0
    D. J11.89

27. **Which code would you use for a diagnosis of viral pneumonia, unspecified?**
    A. J12.9
    B. J18.9
    C. J20.9
    D. J22

28. **What is the ICD-10-CM code for encounter for routine child health examination without abnormal findings?**
    A. Z00.121
    B. Z00.129
    C. Z00.00
    D. Z00.5

29. **Which ICD-10-CM code applies to cellulitis of the left lower limb?**
    A. L03.111
    B. L03.115
    C. L03.116
    D. L03.119

30. **The ICD-10-CM code for obstructive sleep apnea (adult) (pediatric) is:**
    A. G47.30
    B. G47.20
    C. G47.33
    D. G47.39

31. **What is the ICD-10-CM code for gastroenteritis, unspecified?**
      A. K52.9
      B. K51.90
      C. K55.0
      D. K58.9

32. **Which code is used for a diagnosis of acute myocardial infarction, unspecified?**
      A. I21.3
      B. I21.9
      C. I22.0
      D. I25.10

33. **The ICD-10-CM code for epilepsy, unspecified, not intractable, without status epilepticus is:**
      A. G40.909
      B. G40.901
      C. G40.219
      D. G40.299

34. **Which code applies to bacterial pneumonia, unspecified?**
      A. J18.9
      B. J15.9
      C. J13
      D. J18.2

35. **What is the ICD-10-CM code for osteoarthritis of the knee, unspecified?**
      A. M17.10
      B. M19.90
      C. M16.0
      D. M17.9

36. **What code would you assign for dehydration?**
      A. E86.0
      B. E85.9
      C. E87.6
      D. E86.9

37. **Which ICD-10-CM code is used for dysphagia, unspecified?**
      A. R13.10

B. R13.11
C. R13.19
D. R13.12

38. **The ICD-10-CM code for bipolar disorder, unspecified, is:**
    A. F31.9
    B. F32.9
    C. F33.2
    D. F34.0

39. **Which code would be used for an encounter for screening for COVID-19?**
    A. Z11.59
    B. Z20.828
    C. Z11.52
    D. Z13.9

40. **What is the ICD-10-CM code for an abscess of the left foot?**
    A. L03.119
    B. L02.612
    C. L02.619
    D. L03.116

41. **What is the ICD-10-CM code for uncomplicated, type 1 diabetes mellitus?**
    A. E11.9
    B. E10.9
    C. E11.65
    D. E08.9

42. **Which ICD-10-CM code is used for heart failure, unspecified?**
    A. I50.1
    B. I50.9
    C. I51.7
    D. I10

43. **What is the ICD-10-CM code for asthma, unspecified, uncomplicated?**
    A. J45.909
    B. J45.901

C. J44.9
D. J43.9

44. The ICD-10-CM code for contact dermatitis due to poison ivy is:
   A. L23.5
   B. L24.5
   C. L25.5
   D. L30.5

45. Which ICD-10-CM code would you use for acute appendicitis with generalized peritonitis?
   A. K35.2
   B. K36
   C. K35.3
   D. K35.9

46. What is the ICD-10-CM code for chronic viral hepatitis C without hepatic coma?
   A. B18.2
   B. B18.9
   C. B19.20
   D. B17.10

47. Which code is used for benign prostatic hyperplasia with lower urinary tract symptoms?
   A. N40.0
   B. N40.1
   C. N41.9
   D. N39.0

48. What ICD-10-CM code would you assign for nausea with vomiting?
   A. R11.0
   B. R11.2
   C. R11.10
   D. R10.9

49. The ICD-10-CM code for unspecified anemia is:
   A. D64.9
   B. D50.9
   C. D62
   D. D51.9

50. **Which ICD-10-CM code applies to diverticulitis of the large intestine without perforation or abscess?**
    A. K57.90
    B. K57.30
    C. K58.1
    D. K59.00

51. **The ICD-10-CM code for glaucoma, unspecified, is:**
    A. H40.9
    B. H42
    C. H43.3
    D. H40.89

52. **What code is assigned for hyperthyroidism without thyrotoxic crisis or storm?**
    A. E05.0
    B. E05.9
    C. E06.3
    D. E04.9

53. **Which ICD-10-CM code would you use for a diagnosis of chronic tonsillitis?**
    A. J03.90
    B. J35.01
    C. J36
    D. J04.0

54. **The ICD-10-CM code for acute sinusitis, unspecified, is:**
    A. J32.9
    B. J01.90
    C. J01.0
    D. J33.0

55. **Which ICD-10-CM code is used for alcoholic cirrhosis of the liver without ascites?**
    A. K74.6
    B. K70.30
    C. K76.0
    D. K71.50

56. **What is the ICD-10-CM code for obesity due to excess calories?**
    A. E66.9

B. E66.01
C. E66.1
D. E66.8

57. Which code is used for cholelithiasis with acute cholecystitis?
   A. K80.00
   B. K81.0
   C. K82.1
   D. K83.9

58. The ICD-10-CM code for generalized anxiety disorder is:
   A. F40.9
   B. F41.1
   C. F43.1
   D. F42.9

59. Which code represents osteomyelitis, unspecified?
   A. M86.9
   B. M89.8
   C. M85.0
   D. M84.9

60. What is the ICD-10-CM code for malignant neoplasm of the right lung, unspecified?
   A. C34.91
   B. C34.90
   C. C34.80
   D. C34.81

61. What is the ICD-10-CM code for a patient with chronic sinusitis, unspecified?
   A) J32.9
   B) J32.1
   C) J32.0
   D) J01.90

62. Which ICD-10-CM code is used for a patient with asthma, mild intermittent?
   A) J45.909
   B) J45.20
   C) J45.21
   D) J45.901

248

63. What is the correct ICD-10-CM code for a patient diagnosed with hypertension, malignant?
   A) I11.9
   B) I10
   C) I13.0
   D) I10.9

64. Which ICD-10-CM code is assigned for a fracture of the left wrist, initial encounter for closed fracture?
   A) S52.001A
   B) S52.502A
   C) S52.511A
   D) S52.502D

65. What is the ICD-10-CM code for a patient with type 2 diabetes mellitus with diabetic peripheral angiopathy?
   A) E11.9
   B) E11.51
   C) E10.51
   D) E11.59

66. What is the ICD-10-CM code for anxiety disorder due to a medical condition?
   A) F41.9
   B) F41.0
   C) F43.23
   D) F43.22

67. Which code represents chronic rhinosinusitis with nasal polyps?
   A) J32.9
   B) J33.0
   C) J34.2
   D) J32.3

68. What is the ICD-10-CM code for a patient with osteoporosis without current pathological fracture?
   A) M80.00
   B) M81.0
   C) M81.8
   D) M80.88

69. Which ICD-10-CM code is used for a patient with a malignant neoplasm of the colon, unspecified?
   A) C18.9
   B) C19.9
   C) C18.0
   D) C20.9

70. What is the ICD-10-CM code for a patient with recurrent urinary tract infections?
   A) N39.0
   B) N30.91
   C) N30.9
   D) N39.2

71. What is the ICD-10-CM code for a patient diagnosed with type 1 diabetes mellitus with ketoacidosis?
   A) E10.9
   B) E10.10
   C) E10.65
   D) E11.10

72. Which ICD-10-CM code is used for a patient with gout, unspecified?
   A) M10.00
   B) M10.10
   C) M10.9
   D) M10.03

73. What is the correct ICD-10-CM code for a patient with chronic fatigue syndrome?
   A) G93.3
   B) F48.0
   C) R53.82
   D) G93.89

74. Which ICD-10-CM code represents a patient with severe allergic rhinitis due to pollen?
   A) J30.1
   B) J30.2
   C) J30.9
   D) J30.5

75. What is the ICD-10-CM code for a patient with heart failure due to ischemic heart disease?
   A) I50.1
   B) I50.9
   C) I11.0
   D) I13.0

76. Which ICD-10-CM code is assigned for a patient with hyperthyroidism with goiter?
   A) E05.9
   B) E05.0
   C) E05.81
   D) E04.1

77. What is the ICD-10-CM code for a patient with chronic pain syndrome?
   A) G89.4
   B) R52.2
   C) R52.0
   D) G89.0

78. Which code represents a diagnosis of chronic hepatitis B without hepatic coma?
   A) B18.2
   B) B18.9
   C) B19.20
   D) B17.10

79. What is the ICD-10-CM code for a patient with acute appendicitis without peritonitis?
   A) K35.1
   B) K35.2
   C) K35.3
   D) K35.9

80. Which ICD-10-CM code is used for a patient with a malignant neoplasm of the breast, unspecified?
   A) C50.919
   B) C50.92
   C) C50.211
   D) C50.811

81. What is the ICD-10-CM code for a patient with chronic obstructive pulmonary disease (COPD) with acute exacerbation?
   A) J44.1
   B) J44.9
   C) J44.0
   D) J43.9

82. Which ICD-10-CM code is used for a patient with tension-type headache?
   A) G44.1
   B) G43.909
   C) G44.2
   D) G44.3

83. What is the correct ICD-10-CM code for a patient diagnosed with vitamin D deficiency?
   A) E55.9
   B) E55.1
   C) E55.0
   D) E55.2

84. Which ICD-10-CM code represents a patient with stage 1 pressure ulcer?
   A) L89.119
   B) L89.000
   C) L89.101
   D) L89.111

85. What is the ICD-10-CM code for a patient with chronic kidney disease, stage 2?
   A) N18.2
   B) N18.3
   C) N18.1
   D) N18.4

86. Which ICD-10-CM code is assigned for a patient with osteoarthritis of the right hip?
   A) M16.10
   B) M16.11
   C) M16.12

D) M19.90

87. What is the ICD-10-CM code for a patient with obsessive-compulsive disorder?
   A) F42.0
   B) F42.9
   C) F42.1
   D) F42.2

88. Which code represents a diagnosis of malignant neoplasm of the prostate, unspecified?
   A) C61
   B) C62.9
   C) C61.9
   D) C61.1

89. What is the ICD-10-CM code for a patient with an allergic reaction to insect stings?
   A) T63.4
   B) T63.0
   C) T63.2
   D) T63.1

90. Which ICD-10-CM code is used for a patient with a history of transient ischemic attack (TIA)?
   A) Z86.73
   B) Z86.718
   C) Z86.19
   D) Z86.1

91. What is the ICD-10-CM code for a patient with diverticulitis of the large intestine with perforation?
   A) K57.30
   B) K57.90
   C) K57.21
   D) K57.20

92. Which ICD-10-CM code is used for a patient with chronic pharyngitis?
   A) J31.2
   B) J02.9
   C) J35.0

D) J03.90

93. What is the correct ICD-10-CM code for a patient with hypertension, essential, stage 1?
   A) I10
   B) I11.9
   C) I11.0
   D) I13.10

94. Which ICD-10-CM code represents a diagnosis of acute gastritis?
   A) K29.70
   B) K29.90
   C) K29.60
   D) K29.40

95. What is the ICD-10-CM code for a patient with sleep apnea, unspecified?
   A) G47.30
   B) G47.39
   C) G47.20
   D) G47.31

96. Which ICD-10-CM code is assigned for chronic pancreatitis?
   A) K86.1
   B) K85.9
   C) K85.1
   D) K80.0

97. What is the ICD-10-CM code for a patient diagnosed with essential tremor?
   A) G25.0
   B) G25.2
   C) G25.3
   D) G25.9

98. Which ICD-10-CM code applies to a patient with an acute myocardial infarction of the inferior wall?
   A) I21.9
   B) I21.11
   C) I21.19
   D) I21.01

99. What is the ICD-10-CM code for a patient with chronic bronchitis?
   A) J40
   B) J42
   C) J44.9
   D) J41.0

100. Which ICD-10-CM code is used for a patient with urinary incontinence, unspecified?
   A) R32
   B) N39.3
   C) N39.0
   D) R31.9

ANSWER SHEET

1. **B) E10.9** – Type 1 diabetes mellitus, uncomplicated
2. **B) I50.9** – Heart failure, unspecified
3. **A) J45.909** – Asthma, unspecified, uncomplicated
4. **A) L23.5** – Contact dermatitis due to poison ivy
5. **A) K35.2** – Acute appendicitis with generalized peritonitis
6. **A) B18.2** – Chronic viral hepatitis C without hepatic coma
7. **B) N40.1** – Benign prostatic hyperplasia with lower urinary tract symptoms
8. **B) R11.2** – Nausea with vomiting
9. **A) D64.9** – Anemia, unspecified
10. **B) K57.30** – Diverticulitis of the large intestine without perforation or abscess
11. **A) H40.9** – Glaucoma, unspecified
12. **B) E05.9** – Hyperthyroidism without thyrotoxic crisis or storm
13. **B) J35.01** – Chronic tonsillitis
14. **B) J01.90** – Acute sinusitis, unspecified
15. **B) K70.30** – Alcoholic cirrhosis of the liver without ascites
16. **B) E66.01** – Obesity due to excess calories
17. **A) K80.00** – Cholelithiasis with acute cholecystitis
18. **B) F41.1** – Generalized anxiety disorder
19. **A) M86.9** – Osteomyelitis, unspecified
20. **A) C34.91** – Malignant neoplasm of the right lung, unspecified
21. **B) S72.021A** – Fracture of the right femur, initial encounter for closed fracture
22. **D) B15.9** – Acute viral hepatitis B without delta-agent and without hepatic coma
23. **B) F41.9** – Anxiety disorder, unspecified
24. **B) N18.3** – Chronic kidney disease, stage 3
25. **A) K85.9** – Acute pancreatitis
26. **D) J11.1** – Influenza due to unidentified influenza virus, uncomplicated
27. **A) J12.9** – Viral pneumonia, unspecified

28. **B) Z00.129** – Routine child health examination without abnormal findings
29. **B) L03.115** – Cellulitis of the left lower limb
30. **A) G47.30** – Obstructive sleep apnea (adult) (pediatric)
31. **A) K52.9** – Gastroenteritis, unspecified
32. **B) I21.9** – Acute myocardial infarction, unspecified
33. **A) G40.909** – Epilepsy, unspecified, not intractable, without status epilepticus
34. **B) J15.9** – Bacterial pneumonia, unspecified
35. **A) M17.10** – Osteoarthritis of the knee, unspecified
36. **A) E86.0** – Dehydration
37. **A) R13.10** – Dysphagia, unspecified
38. **A) F31.9** – Bipolar disorder, unspecified
39. **A) Z11.52** – Encounter for screening for COVID-19
40. **B) L02.612** – Abscess of the left foot
41. **B) E10.9** – Uncomplicated Type 1 diabetes mellitus
42. **B) I50.9** – Unspecified heart failure
43. **A) J45.909** – Unspecified, uncomplicated asthma
44. **A) L23.5** – Contact dermatitis due to poison ivy
45. **A) K35.2** – Acute appendicitis with generalized peritonitis
46. **A) B18.2** – Chronic viral hepatitis C without hepatic coma
47. **B) N40.1** – Benign prostatic hyperplasia with lower urinary tract symptoms
48. **B) R11.2** – Nausea with vomiting
49. **A) D64.9** – Unspecified anemia
50. **B) K57.30** – Diverticulitis of the large intestine without perforation or abscess
51. **A) H40.9** – Unspecified glaucoma
52. **B) E05.9** – Hyperthyroidism without thyrotoxic crisis or storm
53. **B) J35.01** – Chronic tonsillitis
54. **B) J01.90** – Unspecified acute sinusitis
55. **B) K70.30** – Alcoholic cirrhosis without ascites
56. **B) E66.01** – Obesity due to excess calories
57. **A) K80.00** – Cholelithiasis with acute cholecystitis
58. **B) F41.1** – Generalized anxiety disorder

59. **A) M86.9** – Unspecified osteomyelitis

60. **A) C34.91** – Malignant neoplasm of the right lung, unspecified

61. **A) J32.9 – Chronic sinusitis, unspecified**

62. **A) J45.909 – Asthma, mild intermittent**

63. **C) I13.0 – Hypertension, malignant**

64. **A) S52.001A – Fracture of the left wrist, initial encounter for closed fracture**

65. **B) E11.51 – Type 2 diabetes mellitus with diabetic peripheral angiopathy**

66. **C) F43.23 – Anxiety disorder due to a medical condition**

67. **D) J32.3 – Chronic rhinosinusitis with nasal polyps**

68. **B) M81.0 – Osteoporosis without current pathological fracture**

69. **A) C18.9 – Malignant neoplasm of the colon, unspecified**

70. **B) N30.91 – Recurrent urinary tract infections**

71. **C) E10.65 – Type 1 diabetes mellitus with ketoacidosis**

72. **C) M10.9 – Gout, unspecified**

73. **A) G93.3 – Chronic fatigue syndrome**

74. **A) J30.1 – Severe allergic rhinitis due to pollen**

75. **C) I11.0 – Heart failure due to ischemic heart disease**

76. **B) E05.0 – Hyperthyroidism with goiter**

77. **A) G89.4 – Chronic pain syndrome**

78. **A) B18.2 – Chronic hepatitis B without hepatic coma**

79. **A) K35.1 – Acute appendicitis without peritonitis**

80. **A) C50.919 – Malignant neoplasm of the breast, unspecified**

81. **A) J44.1 – Chronic obstructive pulmonary disease (COPD) with acute exacerbation**

82. **A) G44.1 – Tension-type headache**

83. **A) E55.9 – Vitamin D deficiency**

84. **A) L89.119 – Stage 1 pressure ulcer**

85. **A) N18.2 – Chronic kidney disease, stage 2**

86. **B) M16.11 – Osteoarthritis of the right hip**

87. **B) F42.9 – Obsessive-compulsive disorder**

88. **A) C61 – Malignant neoplasm of the prostate, unspecified**

89. **A) T63.4 – Allergic reaction to insect stings**

90. **A) Z86.73 – History of transient ischemic attack (TIA)**

91. C) K57.21 – Diverticulitis of the large intestine with perforation
92. A) J31.2 – Chronic pharyngitis
93. A) I10 – Hypertension, essential, stage 1
94. A) K29.70 – Acute gastritis
95. A) G47.30 – Sleep apnea, unspecified
96. A) K86.1 – Chronic pancreatitis
97. A) G25.0 – Essential tremor
98. B) I21.11 – Acute myocardial infarction of the inferior wall
99. A) J40 – Chronic bronchitis
100. A) R32 – Urinary incontinence, unspecified

Chapter 8: Learning and Improving from Practice Tests

Congratulations on completing your practice tests! You've taken significant strides in your CPC exam preparation. It's time to make the most of these practice opportunities and fine-tune your coding skills further. This chapter focuses on learning from your mistakes, identifying areas for improvement, and developing a targeted study plan to enhance your performance.

Detailed Explanations for Practice Test Questions

As you embark on your CPC exam preparation journey, take learning from each practice test you take is crucial. Below, we'll help gain an understanding of correct answers, explain incorrect choices, and unravel the rationale behind coding decisions. Delving deeper into the explanations will enhance your coding knowledge and give you the confidence to tackle challenging scenarios. Remember, every question and its explanation offers an opportunity for growth.

Understanding Correct Answers

As you review your practice test results, pay close attention to the questions you answered correctly. Take the time to understand the rationale behind the correct choices. Examine the specific guidelines or codes that support them. This will reinforce your understanding of coding principles and boost your confidence in handling similar scenarios during the real exam. Remember, the CPC exam evaluates not only your ability to memorize codes but also your comprehension and application of coding guidelines.

Example: Suppose you encounter a question related to coding an office visit with a documented blood pressure reading. Understanding the specific guidelines for code selection is essential. You would need to know that a routine blood pressure reading is not separately billable with an office visit, as it is considered part of the evaluation and management service. The correct answer in this case would be to choose the appropriate office visit code without including the blood pressure reading separately.

Explaining Incorrect Choices

Don't be disheartened by incorrect answers; they offer valuable learning opportunities. Analyze the reasons behind your mistakes and examine the guidelines or concepts you may have misunderstood. Identifying and understanding your errors is an essential step in the learning process. It allows you to make targeted improvements and avoid repeating the same mistakes in the future.

Example: If you encounter a question related to coding a laceration repair, but you mistakenly chose the incorrect code, take a closer look at the specific guidelines for laceration repair coding. Pay attention to the documentation requirements, the number of layers repaired, and any additional procedures performed during the repair. Understanding these guidelines will help you select the correct code in similar scenarios.

Rationale Behind Coding Decisions

Explore the thought process behind each coding decision for ambiguous or challenging questions. Understanding the reasoning behind the correct answer will deepen your coding knowledge and sharpen your critical thinking skills, better preparing you for the varied scenarios you may encounter in the CPC exam.

Example: Suppose you encounter a question about coding an excisional biopsy and are unsure about the appropriate code selection. Take the time to analyze the documentation and understand the differences between excisional and incisional biopsies. Understanding the rationale behind choosing the correct code will enhance your ability to differentiate between similar procedures in future exam questions.

Tips for Efficiently Reviewing Practice Tests

Utilize your time efficiently while reviewing practice tests. Focus on the questions that posed the greatest challenge, and examine their corresponding explanations thoroughly. Organize your review process to prioritize areas that require further attention, maximizing your study efforts.

Example: If you have limited time available for review, start by identifying questions that you answered incorrectly. Begin with these questions to understand why you made the mistakes and how to avoid them in the future. Next, move on to questions that were challenging but where you selected the correct answer. Understanding the thought process behind these questions will reinforce your knowledge and coding skills.

Identifying Areas for Improvement

Identifying areas where you may encounter challenges in your CPC exam preparation is a crucial step toward improvement. By enhanced highlighting areas that need extra attention; you can develop a targeted approach to enhancing your coding knowledge and proficiency. Remember, the journey to becoming a skilled medical coder involves acknowledging areas for growth and committing to continuous improvement.

Analyzing Weak Subject Areas

Take note of subjects or coding areas where you consistently encounter difficulties. These weak spots are prime targets for improvement. Prioritize additional study time and resources to reinforce your understanding of these topics.

Example: If you find that coding for cardiovascular procedures is consistently challenging, dedicate extra study time to understanding the anatomy, common procedures, and coding guidelines specific to this area. Focus on cardiovascular system-related concepts and methods to strengthen your coding knowledge.

Recognizing Common Mistakes

Identify recurring errors in your practice test performance. Understanding these patterns will help you address knowledge gaps and avoid making the same mistakes in the future.

Example: If modifiers of. If you frequently select the wrong modifier for specific services, note the common modifier used in coding scenarios. Review the purpose and appropriate use of each modifier to ensure accurate coding.

Keeping Track of Performance Trends

To ensure you're making progress, track your results over time to observe any improvements or declines. Charting your performance trends will provide insight into your growth and help you evaluate the effectiveness of your study strategies.

Example: Create a performance chart that documents your scores for each practice test or study session. Note any significant improvements or areas that require further attention. Observing your progress visually can motivate you to continue studying and strive for continuous improvement.

Setting Personalized Study Goals

Based on your performance analysis, set specific study goals tailored to your needs. Create a study plan that allocates ample time to focus on areas requiring improvement while maintaining a balance with other topics.

Example: If you find that your knowledge of medical terminology is weaker reinforce than that of other coding areas, and set a specific study goal to enhance your understanding of medical terms. Dedicate a certain amount of study time each day or week to reviewing medical terminology and reinforcing your memory.

Conclusion

By now, you've made significant strides in your CPC exam preparation by utilizing smart study strategies, mastering medical terminology, practicing with mock exams, and learning from your mistakes. Embrace your progress, and remember that every step you take brings you closer to success.

In this chapter, you've explored effective study techniques, mnemonics to aid memorization and strategies for tackling multiple-choice questions. By applying these methods, you've equipped yourself with valuable tools to approach the CPC exam with confidence and competence.

As you embark on the next chapter, we'll delve into frequently asked questions that often arise during CPC exam preparation. From navigating the exam registration process to understanding scoring and certification, this chapter will provide the answers you seek. Whether you have questions about exam logistics, study resources, or specific coding scenarios, we are here to support you on your journey to becoming a certified medical coding professional.

Chapter 8: CPC Exam FAQ

Here, we'll address frequently asked questions (FAQ) about the CPC exam, providing have have have valuable insights to ease any concerns or uncertainties. Let's dive into the most common queries and equip you with the knowledge you need for a successful exam experience.

What is the CPC exam, and who administers it?

The Certified Professional Coder (CPC) exam is a rigorous assessment conducted by the American Academy of Professional Coders (AAPC). It is designed to evaluate your proficiency in medical coding and ensure that you possess the necessary skills to assign codes accurately and adhere to coding guidelines.

What format does the CPC exam follow?

The CPC exam is a multiple-choice test featuring 150 questions. It is divided into two parts: 60 questions on medical terminology, anatomy, and coding guidelines (Section 1), and 90 questions on coding scenarios across various medical specialties (Section 2).

How much time do I have to complete the CPC exam?

You'll be granted 5 hours and 40 minutes to complete the entire CPC exam, including a 10-minute break between Section 1 and Section 2.

What are the passing criteria for the CPC exam?

To pass the CPC exam, you need a minimum score of 70%. To ensure you meet this threshold, you must focus on all areas of medical coding.

How should I prepare for the CPC exam?

Effective preparation involves creating a study plan, allocating sufficient study time, utilizing reputable study resources, and practicing with mock exams. Focused study sessions on challenging topics will enhance your understanding.

Can I use my coding books during the exam?

No, during the CPC exam, you cannot refer to any coding books or external resources. You'll need to rely solely on your knowledge and preparation.

How long does it take to receive CPC exam results?

After completing the exam, you can expect to receive your results within 7 to 10 business days. The AAPC will notify you via email, and you can access your results on the AAPC website.

What happens if I don't pass the CPC exam?

If you don't pass the CPC exam on your first attempt, don't be disheartened. You have two additional opportunities to retake the exam within one year of your original exam date. Utilize the feedback from your first attempt to identify areas for improvement and focus on strengthening those aspects during your study for the retake.

Can I appeal my CPC exam results?

Yes, you have the option to appeal your CPC exam results. If you believe there was an error or discrepancy in the scoring process, you can submit a request for an appeal within 30 days of receiving your exam results.

How can I maintain my CPC certification?

To maintain your CPC certification, you must earn 36 Continuing Education Units (CEUs) every two years. These CEUs can be obtained through various educational activities, conferences, workshops, and webinars offered by AAPC-approved providers.

Is the CPC certification recognized nationally?

Yes, the CPC certification is widely recognized and respected in the healthcare industry. Earning this credential demonstrates your expertise and competence in medical coding, making you a valuable asset to employers and potential job opportunities.

What are the benefits of becoming a certified medical coder?

Becoming a certified medical coder opens doors to a rewarding career in the healthcare industry. As a certified professional, you'll have access to diverse job opportunities, higher earning potential, and a sense of pride in contributing to quality healthcare services.

Can I take the CPC exam online?

As of now, the CPC exam is only offered in a physical testing center. However, AAPC may introduce online proctoring options in the future, so stay updated with their official announcements.

What resources can I use to prepare for the CPC exam?

You can utilize AAPC-approved study guides, coding textbooks, online courses, and practice exams to prepare for the CPC exam. Additionally, joining study groups or seeking guidance from experienced coders can be beneficial.

Are there any prerequisites for taking the CPC exam?

While there are no specific prerequisites for taking the CPC exam, it is recommended that candidates have a foundational knowledge of medical terminology, anatomy, and coding principles before attempting the exam.

Can I retake the CPC exam if I fail?

Yes, you can retake the CPC exam up to three times within one year of your original exam date. However, you must wait a minimum of 30 days between each attempt.

What is the best way to manage exam-related stress?

Exam stress is common, but there are ways to manage it effectively. Prioritize self-care, practice relaxation techniques, maintain a balanced study schedule, and stay positive throughout your exam preparation.

Are there any test-taking strategies I should know about?

Yes, implementing test-taking strategies can significantly impact your performance. Read each question carefully, eliminate obviously incorrect answers, and allocate your time wisely during the exam.

Can I use a calculator during the CPC exam?

Yes, you can use a basic calculator during the CPC exam to assist with calculations.

How long is the CPC certification valid?

Once you earn your CPC certification, it remains valid for two years. As mentioned earlier, to maintain your certification, you must accumulate the required CEUs within this period.

Conclusion

We hope you've found the answers to these common questions helpful in preparing for the CPC exam. Remember, the journey to becoming a certified medical coder may seem daunting at times, but with dedication and persistence, you can achieve your goal.

As you embark on your exam preparation, keep in mind that each candidate's experience is unique, and it's okay to encounter challenges along the way. Embrace the learning process and view each obstacle as an opportunity to grow and improve your skills.

Utilize the study tips, test-taking strategies, and practice exams provided in this book to build your confidence and knowledge. Engage in focused study sessions, take advantage of study groups, and don't hesitate to seek help from experienced coders or mentors.

Maintaining a positive mindset and staying committed to your goals will make a significant difference in your exam performance. Remember that the CPC exam is a stepping stone to a rewarding career in the healthcare industry, and obtaining this certification opens doors to a multitude of opportunities.

Lastly, believe in yourself and your abilities. You've come this far in your journey, and you have what it takes to succeed. Keep pushing forward, stay focused, and know that your hard work will pay off in the end.

Conclusion

Here we are at last, at the final chapter of this comprehensive guide to the CPC exam! Throughout this book, we've covered essential topics to prepare you for success in the medical billing and coding profession and equip you with the necessary knowledge and skills to excel in the CPC exam. Let's take a closer look at the key points we've explored and delve deeper into each section to reinforce your understanding.

First, we examined the CPC exam and the medical billing and coding profession in depth. You learned about the importance of medical coders, the complexities of the job, and the extensive licensing requirements. By now, you should grasp the significance of accurate medical coding in ensuring proper reimbursement for healthcare providers and facilitating efficient healthcare operations.

Next, we delved into the reasons why you should consider a career as a medical billing coder. From the rewarding nature of the profession to the potential for job stability and growth, becoming a certified medical coder opens doors to numerous opportunities in the healthcare industry.

We also provided a comprehensive overview of the CPC exam, including the format, content areas, and time allocation. Understanding the exam structure is vital as it allows you to strategize your study plan effectively and allocate sufficient time to each section.

To prepare you for success, we offered smart study strategies tailored to CPC exam preparation. You've learned the importance of creating a study plan, setting realistic goals, and practicing with mock exams to identify areas for improvement. This section also explored various memory-enhancing techniques, such as utilizing mnemonics, repetition, and practical application. These techniques will strengthen your ability to retain information and recall essential medical terms and concepts during the exam.

We focused on challenging subjects, including anatomy and physiology fundamentals, coding guidelines, medical billing, and ethical considerations. Understanding these complex topics is vital for accurate coding and billing practices.

By now, you should also understand test-taking strategies to approach the exam with confidence and efficiency. We also offered extensive practice tests to evaluate your knowledge and readiness for the actual exam. Practicing with real exam-like questions enhances your familiarity with the format and content, preparing you for any surprises on exam day.

Finally, we addressed common queries and concerns related to the CPC exam, providing clarity and guidance to alleviate any apprehensions.

Now that you've completed this comprehensive guide, you're well-equipped to tackle the CPC exam with confidence and proficiency. Remember, success in the medical billing and coding profession is a journey that requires continuous learning and dedication. As you embark on this fulfilling career, embrace challenges as opportunities for growth, and stay committed to enhancing your skills.

The CPC certification serves as a testament to your expertise and opens doors to a rewarding career in the healthcare industry. Congratulations on your commitment to becoming a certified medical coder, and we wish you all the best in your future endeavors!

CONTACT THE AUTHOR

I always strive to make this guide as comprehensive and helpful as possible, but there's always room for improvement. If you have any questions, suggestions, or feedback, I would love to hear from you. Hearing your thoughts helps me understand what works, what doesn't, and what could be made better in future editions.

To make it easier for you to reach out, I have set up a dedicated email address:

✉ epicinkpublishing@gmail.com

Feel free to email me for:

- Clarifications on any topics covered in this book

- Suggestions for additional topics or improvements

- Feedback on your experience with the book

Your input is invaluable. I read every email and will do my best to respond in a timely manner.

Thank you once again for entrusting me with a part of your educational journey.

Best wishes

Medical Terminology Bible

The Simplified Guide to learn medical terms for Medicine Studends, Coders and Healthcare Professions - Get a High-Paying, Rewarding Career – Workbook Included

Contents

"Medicine is a tricky language, but we're here to help you speak it with confidence." — Sir William Osler

The healthcare field is confusing enough, but the technical language can make even straightforward topics more difficult to understand. Medical terms, abbreviations, and acronyms can be confusing, even for the most eager learners. If you're thinking of becoming a medical biller or becoming a healthcare professional, the complex language can be intimidating. This book is your guide to making sense of the complicated words and phrases you'll encounter in healthcare.

Why Are Medical Terms So Confusing?

Have you ever wondered why medical terms are so hard to understand? It may seem arbitrary, but many of these terms have been around for centuries, and often come from different languages and fields. The people who created these terms wanted to be very specific, so they made up new words that may sound similar or are very long. Even today, scientists invent new words for new treatments and discovers, which can make medical terminology even more confusing.

The Importance of Understanding Medical Terminology

Knowing medical terminology is crucial for a career in healthcare. Whether you're a medical biller or a future healthcare worker, understanding these terms is important for many reasons. For medical billers, understanding medical terminology is essential for choosing the correct codes right so providers are paid correctly. Future healthcare workers will need to be able to communicate with other professionals when discussing patient symptoms and treatment options.

How This Book Will Help You

This book will help you understand medical terminology and make it easy to learn and use. Here's what you can expect in the following chapters:

Simple and Easy-to-Understand: We've made sure that the information in this book is easy to understand. We explain things in a simple way and give relatable examples that illustrate each point. With this book, you won't feel lost or overwhelmed by complicated explanations.

Practice Makes Perfect: We believe that the best way to learn is by doing. That's why we've included exercises and real-life situations for you to practice what you've learned. Applying the knowledge you've gained will help you become more confident and skilled in using medical terms.

Everything You Need to Know: This comprehensive book will cover all the important topics you'll come across in healthcare, including body parts and diseases, treatments and tests. And if you ever need to look up a term, our glossary is there to help you find what you need.

Understanding the Context: Medical terms don't exist in a vacuum. They have a history and a reason behind their use. We'll explore the origins and meanings of terms, so you'll understand why they're used, which can help you recall them later.

Tips and Tricks: Memorizing all those words might seem impossible, but we have tips and tricks to make it easier. We'll share memory aids and simple techniques that will help you remember terms so you always have them at your fingertips.

Study Resources: This book comes with helpful study guides, including printable flash cards you can use to build your medical vocabulary. These cards feature some of the most common words you'll run across in the medical field, whether you're becoming a healthcare provider or using our previous book, *Medical Billing and Coding for Beginners*, to launch a new career.

Conclusion

So, get ready to unravel the mysteries of medical terminology. This book is your key to understanding the language of healthcare. Remember, learning medical terms takes time and practice. But with this guide in your hands, you'll soon be speaking the language of medicine with confidence.

BONUS CONTENT

Don't forget to enjoy the free bonuses at the end of this book! Check the last pages!

Enjoy.

P.S. Don't forget to leave a honest review or rating! It takes less than 30 seconds and it is very helpful for us!

"The life so short, the craft so long to learn." — Hippocrates

Welcome to the fascinating world of medical terminology! In this chapter, we will work on unraveling the language that underpins the field of medicine. Medical terminology serves as the foundation of communication in healthcare, enabling accurate documentation, effective patient care, and precise coding and billing processes. While it may seem dense and difficult at first, understanding the logic behind medical language will help make the system easier to understand. Let's dive in and discover the basic structure of medical terms that forms the backbone of this specialized language.

Why Medical Terminology Is Necessary

Medical terminology may be harder to understand than natural language, but it's essential to be as specific as possible. Imagine a world where healthcare professionals couldn't understand each other's jargon. Without this common language, medical providers couldn't discuss patient care or create functioning medical systems. The terminology provides a standardized vocabulary that allows healthcare professionals to communicate clearly and accurately.

Using the correct terms when describing medical conditions, procedures, or treatments ensures clarity and avoids misunderstandings. This clarity is crucial not only for healthcare providers but also for coding and billing processes. Medical billing codes that correspond to the exact treatment patients received ensure that doctors are compensated fairly. It's also important for compliance with regulations and keeps financial systems at hospitals flowing smoothly.

The Basics of Medical Terminology

To understand medical terminology, you first need to grasp its fundamental elements. Medical terms are often derived from Latin and Greek roots, as these languages have long served as the foundation of scientific and medical knowledge. Knowing a little etymology, the study of word origins will help you decipher some of this seemingly strange language.

Prefixes

You've probably noticed that medical terms tend to be long. That's because each word consists of several word elements, including prefixes, root words, suffixes, and combining forms. Prefixes are small elements that are added to the beginning of a word, modifying its meaning. For example, "hypo-" means "under" or "below," so "hypotension" refers to low blood pressure, and "hypothermia" means a person's body temperature is low.

Below are some of the most common prefixes you might come across when studying to work in healthcare or medical billing and coding:

- **(an-):** Meaning "without" or "lack of." For example, "aphasia" refers to the loss of ability to understand or express speech.
- **Anti—denoting "against" or "opposite." An antibiotic** is a substance used to kill or inhibit the growth of bacteria.
- **Bi-:** Referring to "two" or "both." "Bilateral" indicates involvement or occurrence on both sides of a patient's organ or body.
- **Brady-:** Signifying "slow" or "slowness." "Bradycardia" refers to an abnormally slow heart rate.
- **Dys-:** Indicating "difficult," "painful," or "impaired." "Dyspnea" refers to difficulty in breathing.
- **Hyper—Means "excessive" or "above normal." Hypertension** is high blood pressure.
- **Hypo-:** Denoting "low" or "below normal." "Hypoglycemia" refers to low blood sugar levels.
- **Inter-:** Signifying "between" or "among." "Interstitial" refers to the space between cells or tissues.
- **Intra—Refers to "within" or "inside." Intravenous** denotes administering medication directly into a vein.
- **Macro-:** Indicating "large" or "enlarged." "Macrocephaly" refers to an abnormally large head.

- **Micro-:** Meaning "small" or "tiny." "Microscopic" refers to objects or structures that are not visible to the naked eye.
- **Neo-:** Denoting "new" or "recent." "Neonatal" refers to the period shortly after birth.
- **Pan-:** Signifying "all" or "entire." "Pancytopenia" refers to a decrease in all blood cell types.
- **Poly-:** Referring to "many" or "multiple." "Polyuria" is the excessive production of urine.
- **Post-:** Indicating "after" or "behind." "Postoperative" refers to the period following a surgical procedure.
- **Pre-:** Denoting "before" or "prior to." "Prenatal" refers to the time before birth.
- **Pro-:** Signifying "before" or "in favor of." "Prophylaxis" refers to preventive treatment.
- **Re-:** Meaning "again" or "back." "Relapse" refers to the return of a disease or symptom after improvement.
- **Sub-:** Indicating "below" or "under." "Subcutaneous" refers to something beneath the skin.
- **Super-:** Denoting "above" or "excessive." "Superior" refers to something located above or higher in position.
- **Syn-:** Referring to "together" or "united." "Syndrome" refers to a group of symptoms occurring together.
- **Tachy-:** Indicating "fast" or "rapid." "Tachycardia" refers to an abnormally fast heart rate.
- **Trans-:** Signifying "across" or "through." "Transplant" refers to the transfer of an organ from one person to another.
- **Uni-:** Denoting "one" or "single." "Unilateral" indicates involvement or occurrence on one side.
- **Xeno-:** Referring to "foreign" or "from another species." "Xenotransplantation" is the transplantation of organs or tissues between different species.

Root Words

The main part of a medical term, and the element that provides the core meaning, is the root words. For instance, "cardi-" refers to the heart, so "cardiology" is the study of the heart. Root words are typically based on Greek or Latin words, and often refer to organs, systems, or other parts of the body. Below are some of the most common root words you'll find in the medical field.

- **Cardi-:** Referring to the "heart." For example, "cardiology" is the study of the heart and its diseases.
- **Derm-:** Denoting the "skin." "Dermatology" is the medical specialty that focuses on the skin and its disorders.
- **Gastr-:** Indicating the "stomach." "Gastritis" refers to inflammation of the stomach lining.
- **Hepat-:** Signifying the "liver." "Hepatitis" is inflammation of the liver.
- **Nephro-:** Meaning the "kidney." "Nephritis" refers to inflammation of the kidneys.
- **Neuro-:** Denoting the "nervous system." "Neurology" is the branch of medicine that deals with the nervous system.
- **Osteo-:** Referring to "bone." "Osteoporosis" is a condition characterized by weak and brittle bones.
- **Pulmon-:** Indicating the "lungs." "Pulmonary" relates to the lungs or their function.
- **Gastro-:** Denoting the "stomach" or "gastrointestinal tract." "Gastroenteritis" is inflammation of the stomach and intestines.
- **Cardio-:** Signifying the "heart" or "heart-related." "Cardiogram" refers to a record or graph of the electrical activity of the heart.
- **Rhin-:** Referring to the "nose." "Rhinoplasty" is a surgical procedure to reshape the nose.
- **Hemo-:** Denoting "blood." "Hemoglobin" is a protein in red blood cells that carries oxygen.
- **Ophthalm-:** Referring to the "eye." "Ophthalmology" is the branch of medicine that deals with the study and treatment of eye disorders.

281

- **Arthr-:** Denoting the "joint." "Arthritis" is inflammation of one or more joints.
- **Myo-:** Referring to "muscle." "Myocardium" is the muscular tissue of the heart.
- **Cerebr-:** Indicating the "brain." "Cerebral" relates to the brain or its functions.
- **Gynec-:** Denoting the "female reproductive system." "Gynecology" is the branch of medicine that focuses on women's reproductive health.
- **Pod-:** Signifying the "foot." "Podiatry" is the medical specialty that deals with the diagnosis and treatment of foot disorders.
- **Dent-:** Referring to the "tooth." A "Dentist" is a healthcare professional who specializes in oral health and tooth care.
- **Hemat-:** Indicating "blood." "Hematology" is the branch of medicine that deals with the study and treatment of blood disorders.
- **Hepat-:** Denoting the "liver." "Hepatomegaly" refers to an enlarged liver.
- **Osteo—Refers to "bone." Osteopathy** is a branch of medicine that focuses on treating musculoskeletal disorders.

Suffixes

Suffixes are added at the end of a word and often indicate a condition, procedure, or disease. Understanding the suffixes below will help make medical terminology less dense and confusing.

-itis: As we've already mentioned, the suffix "-it is" denotes inflammation. For example, "appendicitis" refers to inflammation of the appendix.

-osis: Indicating a "condition" or "abnormal state." For example, "narcosis" refers to the condition of being unconscious, usually caused by medication.

-ectomy: Referring to "surgical removal" or "excision." "Appendectomy" is the surgical removal of the appendix.

-oma: Signifying a "tumor" or "mass." "Melanoma" refers to a type of skin cancer.

-logy: Denoting the "study" or "science" of a specific subject. "Cardiology" is the study of the heart and its diseases.

-scopy: Indicating a "visual examination" or "inspection." "Endoscopy" refers to a procedure that uses a flexible tube with a light and camera to visualize internal organs.

-graphy: Referring to "recording" or "imaging." "Mammography" is a diagnostic imaging technique used to examine the breast tissue.

-plasty: Signifying "surgical repair" or "reconstruction." "Rhinoplasty" refers to a surgical procedure to reshape the nose.

-pathy: Refers to anything that can be considered a "disease" or "disorder." "Neuropathy" refers to damage or dysfunction of the nerves.

-emia: Indicating a "condition of the blood." "Anemia" is a deficiency of red blood cells or hemoglobin in the blood.

-otomy: Referring to "surgical incision" or "cutting into." "Tracheotomy" is a surgical procedure that creates an opening in the windpipe to facilitate breathing.

-rrhea: Indicating "discharge" or "flow." "Diarrhea" is the condition of having frequent and loose bowel movements.

-algia: Denoting "pain." "Arthralgia" refers to joint pain, and fibromyalgia is a disease that causes constant pain in the nerves.

-uria Refers to a "condition" or "presence" of a substance in the urine. Proteinuria is the presence of abnormal amounts of protein in the urine.

-genesis: Indicating "formation" or "origin." "Osteogenesis" refers to the formation of bone.

-plasia: Denoting "growth" or "development." "Hyperplasia" refers to an abnormal increase in the number of cells in an organ or tissue.

Understanding the Structure of Medical Terms

Now that we know the components of medical terms, you'll be able to decipher words even if they're unfamiliar to you. All you need to do is break down a word into its individual parts, which will give you a sense of its meaning. For example, the term "dermatitis" can be broken into "derm/a" (skin) and "-itis" (inflammation), so you can tell that it refers to inflammation of the skin.

"Hypo-" (under), "glyc/o" (sugar), and "-emia" (blood condition) can be combined to form "hypoglycemia," which refers to low blood sugar levels. Below are a few more examples of how these word elements combine to create different medical terms, each of which is extremely precise.

- **Cardiogram:** "Cardio" refers to the heart, and "gram" indicates a recording or tracing. Therefore, a cardiogram is a graphical representation of the electrical activity of the heart.

- **Osteoporosis:** "Osteo" relates to bones, and "porosis" denotes a condition of porousness. Osteoporosis is a medical condition characterized by a decrease in bone density, resulting in fragile and brittle bones.

- **Gastroenteritis:** "Gastro" refers to the stomach, "enter" relates to the intestines, and "itis" signifies inflammation. Gastroenteritis is the inflammation of the stomach and intestines, typically causing symptoms like diarrhea, nausea, and abdominal pain.

- **Tachycardia:** "Tachy" means fast, and "cardia" pertains to the heart. Tachycardia is a condition characterized by an abnormally rapid heart rate, typically exceeding the normal resting rate.

- **Nephrolithiasis:** "Nephro" relates to the kidneys, and "lithiasis" indicates the presence of stones. Nephrolithiasis refers to the formation of kidney stones within the urinary system.

- **Bronchitis:** "Bronchi" refers to the air passages in the lungs, and "itis" signifies inflammation. Bronchitis is the inflammation of the bronchial tubes, leading to coughing, chest congestion, and difficulty breathing.

- **Neurology:** "Neuro" pertains to the nerves, and "logy" denotes the study of. Neurology is the branch of medicine that deals with disorders of the nervous system.
- **Dermatologist:** "Dermato" relates to the skin, and "logist" indicates a specialist or practitioner. A dermatologist is a medical professional who specializes in diagnosing and treating conditions related to the skin, hair, and nails.
- **Hematology:** "Hemato" refers to blood, and "logy" denotes the study of. Hematology is the branch of medicine that focuses on the study of blood and blood-related disorders.
- **Arthritis:** "Arthro" pertains to joints, and "itis" signifies inflammation. Arthritis is the inflammation of one or more joints, causing pain, stiffness, and swelling.

Decoding medical terms becomes easier when we grasp the meanings of prefixes, root words, and suffixes. Breaking down complex terms into familiar word elements allows us to decipher their significance and navigate the language of medicine with confidence.

Importance of Terminology in Context

While understanding the basic structure of medical terms is essential, it is equally important to recognize the context in which these terms are used. Medical terminology varies across different medical fields, specialties, and sub-disciplines. Terms that hold specific meanings in one area may have different interpretations in another. Therefore, it's crucial to understand medical terms within their appropriate context.

As you delve deeper into the world of healthcare, you'll encounter specialized terminology related to fields such as cardiology, dermatology, orthopedics, and many more. Each area has its own unique set of terms, reflecting the intricacies and nuances of that particular field. Recognizing these variations ensures accurate communication, prevents misunderstandings, and ensures your medical billing codes are accurate.

Keep in mind that medical terminology can be overwhelming at times, even if you understand the root words, prefixes, and suffixes. Terms may seem long and complex. However, with practice and exposure, you will become more comfortable and proficient in understanding and using medical terminology.

Conclusion

Congratulations! You've taken the first step in your journey to becoming fluent in the language of medicine. In this chapter, we explored the significance of medical terminology and its role in accurate documentation, patient care, and coding and billing processes.

We also delved into the basic structure of medical terms, discussing prefixes, root words, suffixes, and combining forms. By understanding the building blocks of medical terms and how they come together, you now have a foundation for deciphering the meanings behind these complex words.

In the next chapter, we'll dive deeper into some specific medical terms related to anatomy and physiology. Get ready to expand your medical vocabulary so you can approach your new career with confidence.

Introduction to Anatomy and Physiology

Anatomy and physiology form the bedrock of understanding the human body. Anatomy focuses on the structure and organization of body parts, while physiology examines how these parts function and work together. Being able to accurately describe the structures and systems within our bodies starts with understanding what they are and how they work.

Our bodies are a collection of interconnected systems, each with its own unique functions and structures. Keep reading for a breakdown for the systems and the body and a list of some of the key terms associated with each.

The Skeletal System

The skeletal system is made up of bones, joints, and connective tissues that provide support and structure to our bodies. Bones are the hard, dense structures that serve as the framework of our skeletal system. They range from the long bones of the limbs, such as the femur and humerus, to the flat bones like the scapula and skull.

Joints connect bones, allowing our bodies to move without losing flexibility. Ligaments, tough bands of connective tissue, hold bones together at the joints, while tendons connect muscles to bones. For instance, the muscles in your upper back pull tendons that move your shoulder.

Familiarizing yourself with the terminology related to the skeletal system means accurately identifying different bones and understanding their functions. For instance, the cranium is the skull's upper part, protecting the brain, while the clavicle, also known as the collarbone, connects the shoulder and the sternum. The patella, commonly known as the kneecap, is a small, flat bone located in the front of the knee joint.

The Muscular System

The muscular system allows our bodies to move, holds us up, and generates body heat. This system consists of three types of muscles: skeletal, smooth, and cardiac:

- Skeletal muscles, attached to bones via tendons, allow voluntary movements, such as walking or lifting objects.
- Smooth muscles, found in the walls of internal organs and blood vessels, enable involuntary movements, such as the contraction of the digestive tract.
- Cardiac muscles are exclusive to the heart, providing the rhythmic contractions that pump blood throughout the body.

Familiarizing yourself with key terms associated with muscles will help you identify specific groups and accurately describe movements. For instance, the biceps brachii, located in the upper arm, is responsible for flexing the elbow joint, while the quadriceps femoris, located in the front of the thigh, extends the knee joint.

The term myology refers to the study of muscles, while myocytes are the specialized muscle cells responsible for contraction. Essential movements are called flexion, the bending of a joint to decrease the angle between two bones, and extension, the straightening of a joint to increase the angle between two bones.

The Cardiovascular System

The cardiovascular system, comprised of the heart, blood vessels, and blood, is responsible for circulating oxygen, nutrients, hormones, and waste products throughout the body. The heart acts as a muscular pump that propels blood through the network of blood vessels. Arteries carry oxygenated blood away from the heart, while veins return deoxygenated blood back to the heart. Capillaries, the tiniest blood vessels, facilitate the exchange of oxygen and carbon dioxide, as well as other substances, between the blood and body tissues.

The cardiovascular system is complex, so the terminology used to describe it can be complicated. Cardiology is a specialized field that focuses on the study of the heart and its disorders. Many anatomical terms describe the structures of the heart and blood vessels. For example, the atria are the two upper chambers of the heart that receive blood, while the ventricles are the two lower chambers responsible for pumping blood out of the heart.

Other key terms associated with this system include blood pressure, which measures the force exerted by blood against the walls of blood vessels; pulse, the rhythmic expansion and contraction of arteries due to the heartbeat; and circulation, the continuous movement of blood through the body.

Additionally, you'll need to know terms like oxygenation, which refers to the process of oxygen binding to hemoglobin in red blood cells. Perfusion describes the delivery of oxygenated blood to body tissues.

The Respiratory System

The respiratory system is responsible for the exchange of oxygen and carbon dioxide between the body and the environment. It comprises the nose, pharynx, larynx, trachea, bronchi, and lungs. Oxygen from the air is inhaled, while carbon dioxide, a waste product of metabolism, is exhaled. Respiration ensures the oxygenation of body tissues and the removal of waste gases.

Like other systems, the respiratory system also has its own unique terminology. Many terms identify different respiratory structures, such as the nasal cavity, pharynx, and trachea. They also aid in understanding respiratory processes, such as inhalation (breathing in) and exhalation (breathing out). The nasal cavity is the hollow space inside the nose, while the pharynx serves as a passageway for both air and food. The trachea, also known as the windpipe, connects the larynx to the bronchi, allowing air to pass into the lungs.

Alveoli are tiny air sacs within the lungs where the exchange of oxygen and carbon dioxide occurs. The diaphragm, a dome-shaped muscle beneath the lungs, plays a crucial role in breathing by contracting and relaxing.

Understanding these terms will help you better understand the intricate workings of the respiratory system. For instance, during inhalation, the diaphragm contracts and moves downward, creating a vacuum that allows air to be drawn into the lungs.

The alveoli, which resemble clusters of grapes, play a vital role in gas exchange. Oxygen from inhaled air diffuses into the bloodstream through the thin walls of the alveoli, while carbon dioxide, a waste product, moves from the bloodstream into the alveoli to be exhaled.

As we explore the anatomy and physiology of the respiratory system, we gain insights into how our bodies take in vital oxygen and remove waste gases. Understanding the terminology associated with this system enables us to describe its structures, processes, and functions accurately.

The Integumentary System

Your hair, skin, and nails together make up the integumentary system. This system serves as a protective barrier against external factors, regulates body temperature, and provides sensory information. Understanding the terminology associated with the integumentary system will allow you to accurately describe various skin conditions and dermatological procedures.

The skin, the largest organ, is composed of two main layers: the epidermis and the dermis. The epidermis is the outermost layer, acting as a shield against environmental elements and preventing water loss. The dermis lies beneath the epidermis and contains blood vessels, nerve endings, hair follicles, and sweat glands.

Melanin is a key term in the integumentary system. It refers to the pigment responsible for determining skin, hair, and eye color. Melanin is produced by melanocytes in the epidermis and helps protect the skin from harmful ultraviolet (UV) radiation.

Various skin conditions can affect the integumentary system. Eczema, a common inflammatory condition, is characterized by itchy, red, and inflamed patches of skin. Dermatitis, a more general term, refers to skin inflammation that can be caused by irritants, allergens, or underlying medical conditions.

The Digestive System

The digestive system breaks food down into nutrients that the body can absorb. Understanding the terminology associated with the digestive system enables us to describe digestive processes accurately and discuss gastrointestinal conditions.

The digestive system comprises several organs, including the mouth, esophagus, stomach, small intestine, and large intestine. Digestion begins in the mouth, where food is mechanically broken down by chewing, and mixed with saliva. The esophagus transports food from the mouth to the stomach, where it undergoes chemical digestion aided by gastric juices.

Digestive functions, such as the process of breaking down food into smaller components and absorption, the uptake of nutrients into the bloodstream, are fundamental to understanding digestive functions. Peristalsis, the rhythmic contraction of muscles that propels food through the digestive tract, ensures efficient movement along the gastrointestinal system.

Various digestive disorders can impact the normal functioning of the digestive system. Gastritis, for example, refers to inflammation of the stomach lining, while constipation is characterized by infrequent bowel movements and difficulty passing stool. Understanding these terms, as well as others that can be understood by their suffixes and prefixes, is essential for accurately identifying and discussing specific digestive disorders.

The Urinary System

The urinary system, also known as the excretory system, is responsible for eliminating waste products from the body and maintaining fluid balance. This crucial system includes various organs and processes, which can be affected by several different ailments and medical conditions.

Some of the organs of the urinary system include the kidneys, ureters, bladder, and urethra. The kidneys filter waste products from the blood and produce urine, which is then transported through the ureters to the bladder for storage. When the bladder is full, urine is eliminated from the body through the urethra.

To work in healthcare or medical coding, you'll also need to know terms like filtration, the process by which waste products are removed from the blood by the kidneys, and urine, the liquid waste product excreted by the kidneys. Micturition, commonly known as urination, refers to the act of emptying the bladder.

You'll also need to know the terms for common disorders that can affect the function of the urinary system function. For instance, urinary tract infections (UTIs) are common infections affecting the urinary system, while renal failure refers to the loss of kidney function.

The Reproductive System

The reproductive system is one of the most complex and often misunderstood systems in the human body. Accurately describing reproductive processes and discussing common fertility conditions requires an in-depth understanding of complex terms and the system itself.

Males and females have completely different reproductive systems, each composed of different organs that fulfill different processes. In males, the reproductive system consists primarily of the testicles, where sperm production occurs, and the penis, which facilitates sexual intercourse and the release of sperm. The prostate is another organ involved in the production of semen, which transports sperm during intercourse.

The female reproductive system includes the ovaries, which produce eggs, and the uterus, where fertilized eggs implant and develop into embryos. The fallopian tubes connect the uterus to the ovaries, while the vulva is essential for intercourse and allowing semen into a woman's body.

Medical professionals need to understand terms such as fertilization, which is the fusion of sperm and egg. Menstruation is a complex biological process in which the uterus wall is shed in a monthly cycle. A wide range of medical problems and lifestyle issues can interfere with the menstrual cycle and cause fertility issues.

Important terms related to the reproductive system include infertility, the inability to conceive a child, and sexually transmitted infections (STIs), which are infections transmitted through sexual contact.

The Endocrine System

Unlike many other anatomical systems, the endocrine system is dedicated to regular physiological processes throughout the body. This system consists of several different glands, including:

- **Pituitary Gland:** Known as the "master gland," the pituitary gland is a small pea-sized gland located at the base of the brain. It secretes various hormones that regulate the functions of other endocrine glands. The pituitary gland controls growth, reproduction, thyroid function, and the production of hormones by the adrenal glands.

- **Thyroid Gland:** Located in the front of the neck, the thyroid gland produces hormones that regulate metabolism, body temperature, heart rate, and the utilization of energy. It secretes thyroxine (T4) and triiodothyronine (T3), which play a crucial role in maintaining overall cellular metabolism.

- **Adrenal Glands:** Situated on top of the kidneys, the adrenal glands produce several hormones that regulate stress responses, blood pressure, and metabolism. The adrenal cortex, the outer layer of the adrenal glands, releases hormones such as cortisol, which helps manage stress, and aldosterone, which regulates salt and water balance. The adrenal medulla, the inner part of the adrenal glands, releases adrenaline and noradrenaline, which are involved in the body's fight-or-flight response.

- **Pancreas:** Found behind the stomach, the pancreas serves both exocrine and endocrine functions. Its endocrine cells, called islets of Langerhans, produce hormones such as insulin and glucagon, which play a vital role in blood sugar regulation. Insulin helps lower blood sugar levels, while glucagon raises them, maintaining glucose homeostasis in the body.

- **Gonads (Ovaries and Testes):** The gonads, including the ovaries in females and testes in males, are responsible for producing reproductive hormones. In females, the ovaries produce estrogen and progesterone, which regulate the menstrual cycle and support pregnancy. In males, the testes produce testosterone, which is involved in the development of male reproductive organs and secondary sexual characteristics.

These glands work in harmony, releasing hormones that regulate various bodily functions and maintain homeostasis within the body. By understanding the roles of these glands, we can better appreciate the complex interplay of hormones and their impact on overall health and well-being.

Healthcare professionals and medical coders need to understand endocrine terminology to discuss hormonal imbalances and related conditions, such as diabetes, hypothyroidism, and adrenal insufficiency. Additionally, you should know terms like insulin, which regulates glucose levels, and cortisol, a hormone involved in the body's response to stress.

The Nervous System

The nervous system is the body's communication network, transmitting signals between various parts of the body and coordinating essential functions. This complex biological system involves detailed terminology associated with the nervous system and its role in sensory perception, motor control, and cognitive processes.

The central nervous system consists of the brain and spinal cord. The peripheral nervous system, comprising the nerves that extend throughout the body, work in harmony to relay information and coordinate responses.

Key terms related to the nervous system include neurons, specialized cells that transmit electrical impulses, and neurotransmitters, which are chemical messengers that enable communication between neurons.

To accurately discuss neurological conditions and procedures, you'll need to understand terms related to disorders and injuries. For instance, a stroke is a disruption of blood flow to the brain, and epilepsy is a neurological disorder characterized by seizures. Many conditions affect the synapse, the junction between two neurons, and myelin, a protective covering around nerve fibers.

Summing Up

In this chapter, we learned a lot about the world of medical terminology, starting with how these complex terms are made. With the tools provided, you may even be able to figure out the meaning of unfamiliar medical terms yourself.

After learning how prefixes, root words, and suffixes combine to convey meaning. We then explored the terminology of the skeletal, muscular, cardiovascular, respiratory, digestive, urinary, and reproductive systems.

In the next section, we'll wrap up book one by covering some common terms associated with disease and medical disorders. This information will help equip you for a career as a healthcare provider or a medical billing and coding professional.

Any system in the body can develop a disorder, and bacteria and viruses can attack any part of the body. The complexity of these factors means terminology associated with medical conditions and diseases can quickly get confusing and complicated. In this chapter, we'll discuss applying what we've learned so far to discussing medical conditions, disorders, and diseases.

Applying Knowledge of Medical Terminology Structure

As we learned in the last chapter, medical terminology follows a structured framework that enables precise and effective communication. By understanding how prefixes, root words, and suffixes work together, you can understand the meaning of a word, even if you've never heard it before.

This is especially important when discussing disorders, where words might include information about the severity, location, and cause of a medical condition. For instance, arthritis indicates inflammation in the joints, while tendonitis refers to a similar condition affecting the tendons.

Common medical terms can also refer to treatments using this same structure. An angiogram is an X-ray taken of blood or lymph vessels. An angioplasty is a procedure designed to widen blood vessels to increase blood flow. Both words use the root words "angio-," so you know they're referring to blood vessels.

Next, we'll take a deeper dive into deciphering medical terminology that refers to illnesses and disorders.

The Terminology for Different Disorders

Medical terminology provides a comprehensive and organized framework for describing specific conditions within the vast realm of disorders. Below you'll find an overview of some common medical expressions, organized by which biological system they affect.

Cardiovascular Disorders

Cardiovascular disorders affect the heart and blood vessels, so most terms will include the root word "cardio" if the condition affects the heart, or "angio" if discussing blood vessel problems. Examples include:

- **Myocardial infarction:** Commonly known as a heart attack, it occurs when blood flow to the heart muscle is blocked, leading to tissue damage.
- **Atherosclerosis:** The buildup of plaque within the arteries, narrowing and hardening them, potentially leading to heart disease and stroke.
- **Arrhythmia:** An irregular heart rhythm that can cause palpitations, dizziness, or fainting.

Respiratory Disorders

Disorders affecting the lungs and other parts of the respiratory system can stem from infectious diseases or autoimmune conditions. Below are a few of the most common :

Asthma: A chronic respiratory condition characterized by inflammation and narrowing of the airways, leading to recurrent episodes of wheezing, coughing, chest tightness, and shortness of breath.

Chronic Obstructive Pulmonary Disease (COPD): A progressive lung disease that may include chronic bronchitis and emphysema. It obstructs airflow obstruction and makes breathing difficult, and is often accompanied by a persistent cough, excessive mucus production, and decreased exercise tolerance.

Pneumonia: An infection that inflames the air sacs in one or both lungs, typically caused by bacteria, viruses, or fungi. People with pneumonia typically have a fever, cough with phlegm, chest pain, difficulty breathing, and fatigue.

Pulmonary Embolism: Pulmonary embolisms occur when a blood clot (thrombus) travels to the lungs and obstructs the pulmonary arteries. They can cause sudden onset of shortness of breath, chest pain, rapid heartbeat, coughing up blood, and dizziness.

Sleep Apnea: A sleep disorder characterized by recurrent interruptions in breathing during sleep. It occurs when the muscles in the throat fail to keep the airway open, leading to episodes of snoring, gasping, and waking up abruptly due to breathing problems.

Digestive Disorders

Disorders that impact the gastrointestinal tract and the organs involved in digestion are known as digestive disorders. These disorders will typically have root words related to digestive organs, such as "esophageal" or "col-." Below are a few of the most common gastrointestinal conditions you should be familiar with:

- **Gastroesophageal reflux disease (GERD):** A chronic condition that causes stomach acid flows back into the esophagus, triggering heartburn and acid reflux.
- **Ulcerative colitis:** A chronic inflammatory bowel disease that causes inflammation and ulcers in the colon and rectum, often resulting in abdominal pain and diarrhea.
- **Gallstones:** Hardened deposits that form in the gallbladder and can cause abdominal pain, bloating, and jaundice.

Neurological Disorders

Neurological disorders are complex, often life-altering medical issues that affect the brain, spinal cord, nerves, and other parts of the nervous system. Because they impact some of the most complex parts of the human body, terms related to neurological disorders can be complicated. Some common examples include:

- **Alzheimer's Disease:** A progressive brain disorder that impairs memory, thinking, and behavior.
- **Parkinson's Disease:** A neurodegenerative disorder that affects movement, causing tremors, stiffness, and difficulty with coordination.
- **Multiple Sclerosis:** An autoimmune disease that affects the central nervous system, leading to communication problems between the brain and the rest of the body.
- **Epilepsy:** A neurological disorder characterized by recurrent seizures caused by abnormal electrical activity in the brain.

- **Migraine:** A common disorder with a variety of symptoms, including recurrent severe headaches, often accompanied by nausea, vomiting, and sensitivity to light and sound.
- **Amyotrophic Lateral Sclerosis (ALS):** ALS is a progressive disease that affects nerve cells in the brain and spinal cord, leading to muscle weakness, paralysis, and eventually respiratory failure.

While these terms can be complex, understanding the root terms can help make this language more transparent. The prefix "neuro-" is commonly used to indicate a connection to the nervous system, like in the terms "neurological" or "neuropathy."

The root word "encephalo-" refers specifically to the brain, as in "encephalitis," which indicates inflammation of the brain. Another important root word is "myel-" which pertains to the spinal cord. Myelopathy is a disorder affecting the spinal cord.

You should also understand the term "cranio-," which refers to the skull. The cranial nerve refers to the nerves that originate from the brain.

Endocrine Disorders

Disorders of the thyroid, pancreas, and adrenal glands can cause hormonal imbalances and a wide range of medical conditions. Below are a few examples of medical terms you might come across when discussing endocrine disorders.

Diabetes mellitus is a chronic metabolic disorder characterized by high blood sugar levels due to insufficient insulin production or resistance to insulin.

Hyperthyroidism: As the prefix "hyper" indicates, hyperthyroidism means a person's thyroid gland is overactive, producing too many hormones.

Hypothyroidism: This condition is the opposite of hyperthyroidism. Without enough thyroid hormone, patients can experience a wide range of symptoms, including fatigue, weight gain, and depression.

Addison's Disease: This rare condition causes a person's adrenal glands to produce insufficient amounts of cortisol and aldosterone. Patients with

Addison's Disease often experience fatigue, weight loss, and low blood pressure.

Polycystic Ovary Syndrome (PCOS): A hormonal disorder in women that causes enlarged ovaries with small cysts that disrupts the normal balance of hormone, leading to irregular periods, infertility, and other symptoms.

The prefix "endo-" means "within" or "internal," and usually refers to the endocrine system. The root word "crin-" refers to secretion, as in "endocrine," meaning the glands that secrete hormones directly into the bloodstream.

Because many of the glands in the endocrine system create hormones, many of the terms associated with disorders relate to over- or underproduction. The term "hyper-" denotes excessive or high, as in "hyperthyroidism," which indicates an overactive thyroid gland.

By contrast, the prefix "hypo-" signifies deficiency or low levels, as in "hypothyroidism," a condition caused by an underactive thyroid gland. The root word "adrenal" refers to the adrenal glands, while "pancrea-" pertains to the pancreas, an important endocrine organ.

Reproductive Disorders

Both the female and male reproductive systems involve intricate interplay of hormones, and even minor imbalances can cause an array of disorders. Many of these conditions can result in infertility, pain, and long-term health issues. Below are some common terms associated with reproductive disorders:

Erectile dysfunction: Also known as impotence, this refers to the inability to achieve or maintain an erection sufficient for sexual intercourse, often due to underlying physical or psychological factors.

Endometriosis is a condition in which the tissue lining the uterus (endometrium) grows outside the uterus, causing pain, fertility problems, and the formation of scar tissue.

Premenstrual syndrome (PMS): A collection of physical and emotional symptoms that occur in the days or weeks before a woman's menstrual period, including bloating, mood swings, breast tenderness, and fatigue.

Benign prostatic hyperplasia (BPH): A noncancerous enlargement of the prostate gland that commonly occurs in older men, leading to urinary problems such as frequent urination, weak urine flow, and difficulty starting or stopping urination.

Pelvic Inflammatory Disease (PID): An infection of the female reproductive organs, typically caused by sexually transmitted infections, resulting in inflammation, pain, and potential damage to the uterus, fallopian tubes, and ovaries.

Like disorders affecting other systems in the body, the reproductive system has its own set of unique terms and words. "Gonads refer to the primary sexual organs, the tests, and the ovaries. Attaching the "hypo-" prefix results in "hypogonadism," which refers to a decreased production of hormones by the sex glands.

 Another essential root word is "endometrial—" which pertains to the endometrium, the tissue lining the uterus. The prefix "dys—" implies abnormality or impairment, as seen in "dysmenorrhea," which refers to painful menstrual periods. Additionally, the prefix "pre-" indicates before, as in "premature ejaculation," which describes the condition where ejaculation occurs too quickly during sexual activity.

In Conclusion

This chapter covered some common medical terms associated with disorders and diseases. We explored a range of conditions across various body systems and learned how prefixes, root words, and suffices combine to create descriptive medical terminology.

Now that you've reached the end of Book 1, you should understand how medical terms are used and how they relate to different medical conditions.

Of course, this isn't a comprehensive list of medical terms, but more of a sample of how these words are built and how they're used. For a more complete resource, see the glossary in the back of the book. In the next chapter, we'll take a look at some medical terms associated with specifical disciplines in medicine.

The medical field is vast, so many practitioners focus on specific area of the body or a particular medical condition. Many of these specializations have their own terminology for different medical conditions, treatments, and tests. As a healthcare provider or medical billing coder, below are a few terms you might see working with specialists:

Cardiology

Cardiology is the branch of medicine that deals with the study and treatment of the heart. Cardiologists treat a wide range of conditions and have an array of highly specialized tests at their disposal. Here are some common medical terms associated with cardiology:

- **Arrhythmia:** Abnormal heart rhythm.
- **Myocardial Infarction:** Also known as a heart attack, it occurs when blood flow to the heart muscle is blocked, leading to tissue damage.
- **Hypertension:** High blood pressure, a condition that can strain the heart and blood vessels.
- **Atherosclerosis:** The buildup of plaque in the arteries, narrowing the blood vessels and increasing the risk of heart disease.
- **Congestive Heart Failure:** A chronic condition where the heart cannot pump blood efficiently, leading to fluid buildup and other symptoms.
- **Echocardiogram:** A test that uses sound waves to create a detailed image of the heart's structure and function.
- **Stress Test:** A test that measures the heart's response to physical exertion, often done on a treadmill or stationary bike.

Orthopedics

Orthopedics focuses on the musculoskeletal system, which includes bones, joints, ligaments, tendons, and muscles. Orthopedic surgeons repair damaged skeletal structures, while massage therapists might treat sprains and other soft tissue injuries.

Fracture: A broken bone.

Osteoarthritis: A degenerative joint disease characterized by the breakdown of cartilage and bone in the joints.

Sprain: An injury to a ligament, often caused by stretching or tearing.

Scoliosis: A sideways curvature of the spine.

Tendinitis: Inflammation of a tendon, usually due to overuse or injury.

X-ray: A common imaging test that uses small doses of radiation to produce images of bones and joints.

MRI (Magnetic Resonance Imaging): A diagnostic test that uses strong magnets and radio waves to create detailed images of bones, joints, and soft tissues.

Gastroenterology

Gastroenterology focuses on the digestive system, including the esophagus, stomach, intestines, liver, and pancreas. This discipline has a variety of specialized terms, including:

- **Gastritis:** Inflammation of the stomach lining.
- **Gastroesophageal Reflux Disease (GERD):** A chronic condition where stomach acid flows back into the esophagus, causing heartburn and other symptoms.
- **Hepatitis:** Inflammation of the liver, often caused by a viral infection.
- **Colonoscopy:** A procedure to examine the colon and rectum using a flexible tube with a camera.
- **Diverticulitis:** Inflammation or infection of small pouches that can develop in the wall of the colon.
- **Upper Endoscopy:** A procedure that uses a thin, flexible tube with a camera to visualize the upper digestive tract, including the esophagus, stomach, and duodenum.

- **Stool Test:** A test that examines a stool sample for signs of infection, inflammation, or other abnormalities.

Neurology

Neurology deals with disorders of the nervous system, covered in the previous chapter. Neurology is a complex discipline that requires sophisticated imaging and testing equipment, which can be confusing. Below are some of the most common terms you'll come across related to neurology:

- **Magnetic Resonance Imaging (MRI) is a** diagnostic imaging technique that uses strong magnets and radio waves to create detailed images of the brain, spinal cord, and other parts of the body. It helps neurologists visualize abnormalities such as tumors, strokes, and multiple sclerosis lesions.
- **Electroencephalogram (EEG):** A test that records the electrical activity of the brain using small electrodes attached to the scalp. It helps neurologists diagnose and monitor conditions such as epilepsy, sleep disorders, and brain activity abnormalities.
- **Deep Brain Stimulation (DBS):** This treatment involves surgically implanting electrodes in specific areas of the brain and connecting them to a device similar to a pacemaker. The device delivers electrical impulses to the brain to manage symptoms of movement disorders such as Parkinson's disease.
- **Lumbar Puncture (Spinal Tap):** In this procedure, a needle is inserted into the lower back to remove a small sample of cerebrospinal fluid (CSF) for analysis. It helps diagnose various neurological conditions, including infections, autoimmune disorders, and certain types of cancer.
- **Nerve Conduction Study:** A test that measures the speed and strength of electrical signals as they travel through a nerve, aiding in the diagnosis of nerve damage or conditions such as carpal tunnel syndrome.

Dermatology

Treatment of conditions related to the skin, hair, and nails falls under the discipline of dermatology. Knowing the terms below will help you navigate this complex medical field:

Eczema: A chronic inflammatory skin condition characterized by itchy, red skin and dry patches.

Psoriasis is a chronic autoimmune disease that causes the rapid buildup of skin cells, leading to thick, scaly patches.

Melanoma: The most dangerous type of skin cancer, which develops in the pigment-producing cells of the skin.

Acne: A common skin condition characterized by pimples, blackheads, and whiteheads.

Dermatitis: Inflammation of the skin, often causing itching, redness, and swelling.

Biopsy is a procedure for removing a small sample of tissue for examination under a microscope. It aids in the diagnosis of skin conditions and skin cancers.

Dermoscopy is a technique that uses a handheld device with magnification and light to examine skin lesions to aid in the diagnosis of melanoma and other skin conditions.

Gynecology:

Gynecology focuses specifically on the female reproductive system. Many gynecological procedures focus on preventative treatment, but many terms are related to specific medical conditions. Here are some common medical terms you'll come across working in this field:

- **Menopause:** The natural cessation of menstruation and fertility in women, typically occurring around the age of 45 to 55.
- **Pap Smear:** A screening test that involves collecting cells from the cervix to detect early signs of cervical cancer or abnormal cell changes.

- **Ovarian Cyst:** A fluid-filled sac that develops within or on the surface of an ovary, often causing pain or other symptoms.
- **Pelvic Inflammatory Disease (PID):** An infection of the female reproductive organs, often caused by sexually transmitted infections, leading to inflammation, pain, and potential damage to the uterus, fallopian tubes, and ovaries.
- **Hysteroscopy:** A procedure that uses a thin, lighted tube to examine the inside of the uterus, diagnose conditions, and perform treatments.
- **Mammogram:** An X-ray of the breast used for breast cancer screening and detection.

Oncology:

Cancer is a complex disease that warrants its own medical field, oncology. Oncologists diagnose and treat a variety of cancers, and some specialize in specific types of tumors. Below are a few of the terms you might come across when discussing oncology:

- **Carcinoma:** A type of cancer that starts in the epithelial cells, which are the cells that line the organs and tissues of the body.
- **Chemotherapy:** The use of drugs to destroy or slow down the growth of cancer cells.
- **Radiation therapy:** The use of high-energy radiation to kill cancer cells and shrink tumors.
- **Metastasis:** The spread of cancer from one part of the body to another, often through the lymphatic system or bloodstream.
- **Remission:** The absence of signs or symptoms of cancer, indicating a response to treatment.
- **Palliative care:** Care that focuses on providing relief from the symptoms and stress of a serious illness, with the goal of improving the quality of life for patients and their families.

Conclusion:

In this chapter, we explored medical terms associated with specialized fields of medicine, including cardiology, orthopedics, gastroenterology, neurology, and dermatology. Each field focuses on specific areas of the body or specific medical conditions, so each may have terminology specific to that specialization.

In the next chapter, we'll continue our exploration of medical terminology by delving into terms associated with surgical procedures. This is an extensive field with a variety of terms related to tools and procedures. Developing an understanding of these terms will be essential if you're planning on working with surgeons and healthcare providers.

The surgical field is a specialized area of medicine that involves the use of operative techniques to treat diseases, injuries, and other conditions. Within this field, a multitude of medical terms describe various surgical procedures, tools, and anatomical structures. In this chapter, we'll familiarize ourselves with common terms associated with the surgical field, divided into different types: surgical procedures, surgical instruments, and anatomical terms.

Common Surgical Terms

Surgical procedures include a wide range of operations performed to address or diagnose medical conditions. Understanding the terminology associated with surgical procedures is essential for both healthcare professionals and medical billing coders.

Like other medical terms, surgical terms are comprised of root words, prefixes, and suffixes, which together provide insight into the procedure's purpose and characteristics. Understanding the meaning of these linguistic components will help you decipher the specific aspects of the surgery and the structures involved. Let's explore how different suffixes contribute to surgical terms.

Root Words

Root words serve as the foundation of surgical terms, representing the main body part or organ being operated on. For example, the root word "append" in "appendectomy" refers to the appendix, while "mast" in "mastectomy" relates to the breast. Knowing these terms can tell you a great deal about the site of a surgery.

Suffixes

Suffixes in surgical terms provide additional information about the nature and purpose of the surgery. The suffix "-ectomy" signifies the surgical removal or excision of a specific organ or tissue. It's frequently used in surgical terms to describe the removal of a body part. For example, "appendectomy" refers to the removal of the appendix, "tonsillectomy" involves the removal of the tonsils, and "hysterectomy" denotes the removal of the uterus. The "-ectomy" suffix helps identify procedures involving the excision or removal of a targeted anatomical structure.

308

Another common suffix is "-plasty," which indicates the surgical repair, reconstruction, or reshaping of a body part. For instance, "rhinoplasty" refers to a surgical procedure to reshape the nose, "mastopexy" involves lifting and reshaping the breasts, and "dermoplasty" refers to the surgical repair of skin.

You'll also need to know the suffix "-ostomy," which denotes the creation of an opening or passage between an organ and the outside of the body. It is commonly used to describe procedures involving the creation of a stoma. For example, "colostomy" involves creating an opening in the colon, "ileostomy" refers to creating an opening in the ileum, and "tracheostomy" involves creating an opening in the trachea to establish an airway.

Finally, the suffix "-scopy" indicates the use of an endoscope or a minimally invasive instrument to examine a body cavity or organ. These procedures typically involve inserting a thin, flexible tube with a camera or light source into the body. For instance, "colonoscopy" involves the examination of the colon using a colonoscope and "arthroscopy" refers to the visualization of joint conditions. "Laparoscopy" involves using a laparoscope to examine the abdomen.

Prefixes

Prefixes may contribute to the overall meaning of a surgical term. While they may not be as prevalent in surgical terms compared to other medical terms, they can still provide important context.

For example, the prefix "lapar-" in "laparoscopy" refers to the abdomen, indicating that the procedure involves the use of a laparoscope to visualize the abdominal cavity. Other prefixes such as "arthro-" (related to joints) or "gastro-" (related to the stomach or gastrointestinal system) may be present in surgical terms, depending on the procedure and the anatomical structures involved.

Now that you know how surgical terms are constructed, you'll be able to decipher some of these complex terms. First, we'll take a look at some examples of common surgical procedures.

Types of Surgeries

- **Appendectomy:** The surgical removal of the appendix, usually performed in cases of appendicitis, an inflammation of the appendix. An appendectomy is typically performed to prevent the appendix from rupturing and causing a potentially life-threatening infection.

- **Cholecystectomy:** The surgical removal of the gallbladder, often performed to treat gallstones or gallbladder disease. This procedure is commonly done using minimally invasive techniques, such as laparoscopy, which involves making small incisions and using a laparoscope to visualize and remove the gallbladder.

- **Mastectomy:** The surgical removal of one or both breasts, commonly done as a treatment for breast cancer or to reduce the risk of developing breast cancer in high-risk individuals. Mastectomy can involve different techniques, including total mastectomy (removal of the entire breast), modified radical mastectomy (removal of the breast tissue and nearby lymph nodes), or nipple-sparing mastectomy (preserving the nipple and areola).

- **Colon resection:** The surgical removal of a portion of the colon, typically performed to treat conditions like colon cancer, diverticulitis, or inflammatory bowel disease. Colon resection may involve removing a segment of the colon and reconnecting the remaining ends or creating an ostomy, where an opening is made in the abdominal wall to allow waste to pass out of the body.

- **Arthroscopy is a** minimally invasive surgical procedure that uses a small camera (arthroscope) to visualize and treat joint-related conditions, such as torn cartilage or ligament injuries. During arthroscopy, small incisions are made to insert the arthroscope and other surgical instruments, allowing the surgeon to assess and address issues within the joint.

- **Coronary Artery Bypass Grafting (CABG) is a surgical procedure used to treat coronary artery disease. It** involves taking a healthy blood vessel, typically from the leg or chest, and grafting it onto a blocked or narrowed coronary artery to improve blood flow to the heart.

- **Joint Replacement (Arthroplasty):** A surgical procedure that involves replacing a damaged joint with a prosthetic implant. Joint replacement is commonly performed in conditions such as severe arthritis or joint degeneration, providing relief from pain and restoring joint function.

- **Hysterectomy:** A surgical procedure to remove the uterus. Hysterectomy can be performed through various approaches, including abdominal, vaginal, or laparoscopic methods. It may be done for various reasons, such as uterine fibroids, endometriosis, abnormal uterine bleeding, or gynecological cancers.

- **Cataract Surgery is a surgical procedure to remove a cloudy lens (cataract) from the eye and replace it with an artificial intraocular lens. It** is typically performed when vision impairment affects daily activities and quality of life.

- **Roux-en-Y Gastric Bypass:** This is a surgical procedure for weight loss that involves creating a small stomach pouch and rearranging the small intestine to bypass a portion of it. Roux-en-Y gastric bypass restricts food intake and changes the digestion process to aid in weight reduction.

Surgical Instruments and Equipment:

Surgical instruments and equipment play a vital role in performing surgical procedures accurately and safely. Some tools are used in almost every surgery, while others have very specialized functions. Anyone working in surgical rooms will need to have an in-depth understanding of the terms associated with these instruments and pieces of equipment.

- **Scalpel:** A sharp, precision cutting instrument used by surgeons to make incisions during surgical procedures. Scalpels come in various sizes and shapes, allowing for different types of incisions based on surgical needs.

- **Forceps:** Surgical instruments with two blades and a handle used for grasping, holding, and manipulating tissues or objects during surgery. Forceps come in different shapes and sizes and are specialized for specific purposes, such as tissue dissection, clamping blood vessels, or removing foreign bodies.

- **Retractor:** A handheld surgical instrument used to hold back tissues or organs, providing the surgeon with better visibility and access to the surgical site. Retractors come in various designs, including handheld retractors and self-retaining retractors, allowing for optimal exposure to the surgical field.

- **Electrocautery:** A device that uses high-frequency electrical currents to cut through tissues and coagulate blood vessels, minimizing bleeding during surgery. Electrocautery instruments, such as the Bovie electrocautery device, are commonly used to make precise cuts and control bleeding simultaneously.

- **Laparoscope:** A thin, flexible tube with a camera and light source used to visualize the inside of the abdomen or pelvis during minimally invasive surgeries. Laparoscopic procedures involve making small incisions through which the laparoscope and other instruments are inserted, reducing the need for large surgical incisions.

- **Trocar:** A sharp-pointed surgical instrument with a hollow tube used to create access into body cavities or organs during minimally invasive procedures. Trocars are inserted through small incisions to provide a pathway for the insertion of other instruments or the drainage of fluids.

- **Surgical Stapler:** A specialized device used to close wounds or connect tissues during surgery. Surgical staplers are designed to replace traditional sutures and are commonly used in procedures such as gastrointestinal surgeries, thoracic surgeries, and certain types of open surgeries. They provide efficient and secure closure, reducing operating time and promoting faster healing.

- **Hemostat:** A surgical instrument with hinged, scissor-like handles and clamping jaws used to grasp and hold blood vessels or other tissues, enabling the surgeon to control bleeding during procedures. Hemostats come in various sizes and designs, including straight and curved jaws, allowing for optimal accessibility and maneuverability.

Surgical Procedures

Performing surgery involves a variety of techniques, from preparing the patient to ensuring their safety. Understanding terms associated with these techniques will help healthcare professionals provide better care to their patients and allow medical billing coders to ensure their invoices are as accurate as possible. Keep reading to learn a few of the terms commonly used in surgical suites.

- **Incision:** A cut made through the skin and underlying tissues to access the surgical site. The location and length of the incision depend on the specific procedure and the surgical approach chosen.
- **Suture:** A stitch or thread used to hold together the edges of an incision or to repair tissues during surgery. Sutures can be absorbable (dissolve over time) or non-absorbable (require removal after healing).
- **Anesthesia:** The use of medications to induce a temporary loss of sensation or consciousness during surgery, ensuring that patients are pain-free and unaware of the procedure. Different types of anesthesia include general anesthesia (complete loss of consciousness), regional anesthesia (numbing a specific region of the body), and local anesthesia (numbing a specific area).
- **Hemostasis:** The control or stopping of bleeding during surgery, achieved through various techniques such as ligating blood vessels, cauterization, or using hemostatic agents. Maintaining hemostasis is

crucial for ensuring clear visibility and preventing excessive blood loss during surgical procedures.

- **Anastomosis:** The surgical connection of two separate structures, such as blood vessels, intestines, or ducts, to restore or redirect normal flow or function. Anastomosis is commonly performed to bypass blockages, create new pathways, or reconstruct damaged or removed parts of the body.

- **Ligature:** A thread or suture used to tie off a blood vessel or other anatomical structure to stop bleeding or secure tissue during surgery. Ligatures are commonly used in procedures where precise control of blood flow is necessary, such as vascular surgeries or organ transplantation.

- **Drain:** A surgical device or tube used to remove excess fluid or air from a wound or body cavity. Drains are inserted during surgery and are often used to prevent the accumulation of fluid, promote healing, and reduce the risk of infection. They can be temporary or permanent, depending on the patient's needs.

- **Wound Dressing:** Material applied to a surgical incision or wound to protect it, promote healing, and prevent infection. Wound dressings may include adhesive bandages, sterile gauze, foam dressings, or specialized wound care products. They provide a barrier against contaminants, absorb excess fluid, and create a conducive environment for wound healing.

It is important to note that while this chapter provides an overview of common terms associated with the surgical field, the specific terminology used may vary depending on the surgical specialty and procedure. Many specialists also use tools you may not find in most operating rooms.

The dynamic nature of medical technology also means new tools and devices are introduced constantly. To keep up with the rapidly evolving medical field, healthcare professionals in every field should keep up with the latest developments, especially as surgeons begin to use robots, AI, and other sophisticated technologies.

So far, we've covered some basic terms related to some medical specializations and taken a closer look at the terminology of the operating room. Next, we'll continue our deep dive by learning about some of the medical terms associated with pediatrics. Because pediatric medicine is one of the largest fields of medicine, understanding the unique terms used in this discipline is essential for a successful career.

What Is Pediatrics?

Pediatrics is a specialized branch of medicine that focuses on the healthcare and well-being of infants, children, and adolescents. Pediatricians play a vital role in promoting children's health, growth, and development and diagnosing and managing various pediatric conditions.

Treating the conditions unique to young patients means pediatricians often use their own terms for diseases, treatments, and tests. In this chapter, we'll explore a range of medical terms associated specifically with pediatric medicine. These terms are unique to the field of pediatrics and reflect the specialized knowledge and care required to meet the unique needs of young patients.

Terms for Treatments in Pediatric Medicine

Caring for children, infants, and teenagers often means treating diseases and disorders unique to young people. The language of pediatrics includes a variety of treatment approaches tailored to the specific needs of children. Below are some of the terms you might encounter working in the field of pediatrics:

- **Neonatal Resuscitation:** Neonatal resuscitation refers to the medical intervention performed immediately after birth to support and stabilize newborns who are not breathing or experiencing difficulty breathing. This critical procedure involves techniques such as providing positive pressure ventilation, clearing the airway, and administering medications if necessary.

- **Growth Hormone Therapy:** Growth hormone therapy is a treatment approach that involves administering synthetic growth hormone to children with growth disorders, such as growth hormone deficiency. This therapy helps stimulate growth and development, improving a child's height and overall growth trajectory.

- **Immunization:** Immunization plays a crucial role in pediatric medicine by protecting children against infectious diseases. The process involves administering vaccines to build immunity and prevent or reduce the severity of diseases such as measles, mumps, rubella, and polio.

- **Nutritional Counseling:** Nutritional counseling is an integral part of pediatric care, focusing on providing guidance and education on appropriate nutrition for children. Pediatricians provide nutritional counseling to address various issues, including healthy eating habits, weight management, food allergies, and dietary deficiencies.

- **Inhalation Therapy:** Inhalation therapy involves administering medication in the form of a mist or aerosol that is inhaled into the lungs. This treatment is commonly used to manage respiratory conditions such as asthma, bronchiolitis, and cystic fibrosis. Inhalation therapy helps deliver medication directly to the airways, providing targeted relief and improving breathing.

- **Orthopedic Bracing:** Orthopedic bracing is a treatment approach used in pediatric medicine to support and stabilize musculoskeletal conditions. Pediatric orthopedic bracing involves the use of specialized braces, splints, or casts to manage conditions such as scoliosis, clubfoot, or fractures. These devices provide support, help maintain proper alignment, and promote healing and rehabilitation.

- **Rehabilitation:** Rehabilitation plays a crucial role in pediatric medicine, aiding in the recovery and improvement of physical, cognitive, and psychological functions. Pediatric rehabilitation may involve physical therapy, occupational therapy, or speech therapy, as well as specialized programs addressing developmental delays, motor skills, or rehabilitation after surgeries or injuries.

While the treatments mentioned above provide a glimpse into the range of interventions used in pediatric medicine, they represent only a fraction of the comprehensive care provided by pediatricians. These doctors are skilled healthcare professionals who specialize in caring for the unique medical needs of children from infancy through adolescence. Their expertise extends far beyond the treatments mentioned, covering a wide range of conditions and healthcare services.

From preventive care and routine check-ups to diagnosing and managing acute and chronic illnesses, pediatricians play a vital role in ensuring the health and well-being of children. They address various aspects of pediatric medicine, including physical, emotional, and behavioral health.

In addition to the treatments mentioned, pediatricians may also provide services such as allergy management, vaccination schedules, developmental screenings, and guidance on nutrition and growth. Pediatricians are well-versed in identifying and managing common pediatric conditions such as respiratory infections, gastrointestinal disorders, skin conditions, and childhood obesity. They also play a pivotal role in monitoring growth and development, detecting early signs of developmental delays, and providing appropriate interventions.

Common Conditions Treated by Pediatricians

Children have unique medical needs as they develop, and are more vulnerable to a wide range of medical issues. Pediatricians focus on these specific conditions and disorders to help children develop into healthy adults. If you're working with pediatricians in a billing or support capacity, below are some terms you should be familiar with:

- **Pediatric Asthma:** Pediatric asthma is a chronic respiratory condition characterized by recurring episodes of wheezing, coughing, shortness of breath, and chest tightness. It is typically managed with medications to control symptoms and prevent asthma attacks.

- **Developmental Delay:** Developmental delay refers to a condition in which a child lags behind their peers in achieving developmental milestones such as walking, talking, or social skills. Developmental delay can be caused by various factors, including genetic disorders, neurological conditions, or environmental factors.

- **Pediatric Infectious Diseases:** Pediatric infectious diseases are diseases caused by microorganisms such as bacteria, viruses, fungi, or parasites that affect children. Examples include chickenpox, influenza, strep throat, and urinary tract infections. Pediatricians diagnose and treat infectious diseases using appropriate medications and interventions.

- **Congenital Heart Defect:** Congenital heart defects are structural abnormalities of the heart that are present at birth. These defects can range from minor issues to complex conditions requiring surgical intervention or ongoing medical management.
- **Diabetes:** Pediatricians play a critical role in the diagnosis and management of diabetes in children. Pediatric diabetes refers to a condition in which a child's body has difficulty regulating blood sugar levels. Types of pediatric diabetes include type 1 diabetes, an autoimmune condition that requires lifelong insulin therapy, and type 2 diabetes, often associated with obesity and lifestyle factors.
- **Pediatric Mental Health Disorders:** Pediatricians are involved in the identification and management of various mental health disorders in children, including anxiety disorders, attention-deficit/hyperactivity disorder (ADHD), and depression. They collaborate with mental health professionals to provide comprehensive care, which may include therapy, medication management, and support for families.
- **Pediatric Allergies:** Pediatricians diagnose and manage a wide range of allergies in children, including food allergies, environmental allergies (such as pollen or pet dander), and allergic rhinitis. They help determine triggers, develop allergy management plans, and prescribe appropriate medications to alleviate symptoms and prevent allergic reactions.

Pediatricians offer a wide spectrum of care, addressing both the physical and mental health needs of children. From preventive care and routine check-ups to the diagnosis and management of various acute and chronic illnesses, pediatricians play a vital role in ensuring the overall health and well-being of their young patients.

Tools and Tests Used by Pediatricians

In this section, we'll explore the tools and tests commonly used by pediatricians to aid in the diagnosis, evaluation, and monitoring of pediatric conditions. These tools and tests are integral to the practice of pediatric medicine, providing valuable insights into a child's health and helping doctors develop effective treatment plans. Below are a few of the terms medical billing and coders will encounter working with pediatricians.

- **Pulse Oximetry:** Pulse oximetry is a noninvasive test that measures the oxygen saturation level in the blood. Pediatricians use it to assess a child's respiratory function and determine if additional interventions are necessary.

- **Newborn Screening:** Newborn screening involves a series of tests performed shortly after birth to identify genetic, metabolic, hormonal, and functional disorders that may not be apparent at birth. Newborn screening helps detect conditions such as phenylketonuria, cystic fibrosis, and congenital hypothyroidism, allowing for early intervention and treatment.

- **Otoscope:** An otoscope is a handheld instrument used to examine the ear canal and eardrum. Pediatricians use it to assess children's ear health, diagnose ear infections, and identify other ear-related conditions.

- **Growth Chart:** A growth chart is a visual representation of a child's growth over time, typically plotted using height, weight, and head circumference measurements. Growth charts help pediatricians monitor a child's growth trajectory, identify growth issues, and assess overall development.

- **Developmental Screening:** Developmental screening is a series of standardized assessments designed to evaluate a child's development across various domains, including cognitive, motor, communication, social-emotional, and adaptive skills. Pediatricians use developmental screening tools to identify potential delays or concerns in a child's development. These tests help detect early signs of developmental disorders and facilitate early intervention and support.

- **Allergy Testing:** Pediatricians may utilize various allergy tests to identify specific allergens triggering allergic reactions in children. These tests can include skin prick tests, where small amounts of allergens are applied to the skin to check for a reaction, or blood tests to measure the presence of allergen-specific antibodies. Allergy testing assists in diagnosing and managing conditions such as food allergies, environmental allergies, or allergic asthma, allowing for targeted allergen avoidance measures and appropriate treatment plans.

Conclusion:

Pediatricians specialize in providing comprehensive care to children, addressing their specific medical needs, and promoting their overall health and development. By familiarizing ourselves with these medical terms, we can better understand pediatric medicine's unique challenges and interventions.

This knowledge enables effective communication with pediatric healthcare professionals and empowers professionals to provide support and achieve better patient outcomes. In the next chapter, we'll explore medical terms associated gynecology, another complex medical specialty.

Chapter 7: Medical Terminology in Gynecology

As we mentioned early, gynecology is a specialized field of medicine that focuses on the health and well-being of the female reproductive system. Gynecologists play a vital role in providing comprehensive care to women, addressing various gynecological conditions, and promoting women's overall health.

In this chapter, we'll explore a variety of medical terms associated with gynecology. Understanding these terms is crucial in facilitating effective communication between healthcare professionals and patients, ensuring clarity and informed decision-making in women's healthcare.

Terms for Anatomy and Physiology

The Female Reproductive System

The female reproductive system is a complex network of organs and structures that work together to facilitate reproduction. Understanding the medical terms associated with the female reproductive system is essential for developing an advanced understanding of gynecology. Key terms include:

- **Ovaries:** The two almond-shaped organs responsible for producing eggs and hormones, such as estrogen and progesterone.
- **Uterus:** The muscular organ where fertilized eggs implant and develop into a fetus during pregnancy.
- **Fallopian Tubes:** The tubes that transport eggs from the ovaries to the uterus, where fertilization occurs.
- **Vagina:** The elastic, muscular canal that connects the uterus to the external genitalia.
- **Cervix:** The lower part of the uterus that opens into the vagina.

Breast Anatomy

The breasts, though not directly related to reproduction, are an important area of focus in women's health. These organs include several structures that often require the care of a skilled medical professional.

- **Mammary Glands:** The glandular structures within the breasts responsible for milk production.

- **Areola:** The pigmented area surrounding the nipple.
- **Nipple:** The raised projection on the breast through which milk is released during breastfeeding.

Gynecological Conditions and Disorders:

Many medical conditions and disorders are specific to the female body and the reproductive system. Describing these conditions requires specific terminology that can confuse the lay person. Below is an overview of different types of disorders and key terms associated with each.

Menstrual Disorders:

Menstrual disorders can significantly impact a woman's quality of life, resulting in serious pain and making daily life impossible. Understanding the medical terms associated with these conditions is essential for accurate diagnosis and appropriate management. Here are some common menstrual disorders:

- **Dysmenorrhea:** Severe menstrual cramps often associated with pain and discomfort during menstruation.
- **Menorrhagia:** Heavy or prolonged menstrual bleeding beyond normal levels.
- **Amenorrhea:** The absence of menstruation, which may be temporary or permanent.
- **Premenstrual Syndrome (PMS):** A combination of emotional and physical symptoms that occur before the menstrual period.
- **Polycystic Ovary Syndrome (PCOS):** A hormonal disorder characterized by enlarged ovaries with small cysts and hormonal imbalances.

Reproductive System Infections

Infections affecting the female reproductive system can cause discomfort and potentially lead to serious complications, including infertility and long-term tissue damage. Here are some medical terms associated with common reproductive system infections:

- **Urinary Tract Infections (UTIs):** Infections that affect the urinary system, including the bladder and urethra.
- **Vaginitis:** Inflammation of the vagina, often caused by infections or irritants.
- **Pelvic Inflammatory Disease (PID):** An infection of the female reproductive organs, usually caused by sexually transmitted bacteria.
- **Candidiasis:** A fungal infection caused by Candida overgrowth, commonly known as a yeast infection.
- **Bacterial Vaginosis (BV):** An imbalance of bacteria in the vagina that can cause abnormal discharge and odor.

Gynecological Cancers:

Gynecological cancers can be life-threatening if not detected and treated early. This dangerous disease can affect every part of the female anatomy, from the breasts to the reproductive system. Terms associated with gynecological cancers can tell you which part of the body is affected, which can indicate the cause. Below are a few terms associated with gynecological cancers:

- **Ovarian Cancer:** Cancer that develops in the ovaries, often detected at advanced stages due to its asymptomatic nature.
- **Cervical Cancer:** Cancer that develops in the cervix, often caused by persistent infection with high-risk strains of human papillomavirus (HPV).
- **Uterine Cancer:** Cancer that occurs in the uterus, typically detected early due to symptoms such as abnormal vaginal bleeding.
- **Vulvar Cancer:** Cancer that affects the external genitalia, specifically the vulva.
- **Vaginal Cancer:** Cancer that develops in the vaginal lining, typically rare and often associated with other gynecological cancers.

Diagnostic Procedures and Treatments:

Gynecological issues can be difficult to diagnose and treat, especially since many conditions can be traced to a variety of causes. Gynecologists employ a range of specialized diagnostic procedures and treatments to ensure accurate diagnoses, effective management, and optimal outcomes. Let's explore some common tools and tests used in gynecology:

Pap Smear: A screening test that involves collecting cells from the cervix to detect cervical cell abnormalities or precancerous changes.

HPV Testing: A test that identifies the presence of high-risk strains of human papillomavirus, which can lead to cervical cancer.

Hysteroscopy: A procedure that involves inserting a thin, lighted tube through the cervix into the uterus to visualize and diagnose uterine abnormalities or perform surgical interventions.

Laparoscopy: A minimally invasive surgical procedure that uses a small incision and a laparoscope (a thin, flexible tube with a camera) to visualize and diagnose conditions within the pelvic and abdominal cavities.

Contraception

In addition to diagnosing and treating gynecological conditions, gynecologists also play a crucial role in providing contraception and family planning services. They're trained to provide guidance on the various contraceptive options available, considering an individual's unique needs and medical history. While gynecologists have a variety of contraceptive options available, below is an overview of some of the most popular treatments:

- **Oral Contraceptives (Birth Control Pills):** These are hormonal medications taken orally on a daily basis to prevent pregnancy. They contain synthetic hormones that regulate the menstrual cycle and inhibit ovulation.
- **Intrauterine Device (IUD):** An IUD is a small, T-shaped device inserted into the uterus by a gynecologist. It provides long-term contraception and can be either hormonal (releasing progestin) or non-hormonal (made of copper).
- **Contraceptive Implant:** A small rod inserted under the skin by a gynecologist is usually placed in the upper arm and releases hormones to prevent pregnancy for several years.

- **Depo-Provera (Birth Control Shot):** This is an injectable contraceptive administered by a gynecologist every three months. It contains a progestin hormone that prevents ovulation and thickens cervical mucus.
- **Barrier Methods:** These include condoms (male or female) and diaphragms. Condoms are worn over the penis or inserted into the vagina to prevent sperm from reaching the egg. Diaphragms are dome-shaped devices inserted into the vagina to cover the cervix and block sperm.

Minimally Invasive Procedures:

Minimally invasive procedures have transformed gynecological care by providing alternative approaches that minimize the impact on patients' bodies. These procedures offer several advantages, including reduced pain, shorter hospital stays, faster recovery times, and improved cosmetic outcomes. Gynecologists use state-of-the-art equipment and specialized techniques to perform these procedures with precision. Here are some commonly performed minimally invasive procedures in gynecology:

- **Hysteroscopy:** This procedure involves the insertion of a thin, lighted tube called a hysteroscope through the vagina and cervix to examine the inside of the uterus. It allows gynecologists to diagnose and treat conditions such as abnormal uterine bleeding, polyps, fibroids, and uterine septum.
- **Laparoscopy:** Laparoscopy is a minimally invasive surgical procedure that uses a laparoscope—a thin, flexible tube with a camera and light—to visualize and operate within the abdomen and pelvis. Gynecologists often utilize laparoscopy for diagnosing and treating various conditions, including endometriosis, ovarian cysts, ectopic pregnancies, and pelvic pain.
- **Endometrial Ablation:** This minimally invasive procedure involves the removal or destruction of the uterine lining (endometrium) to manage heavy or abnormal uterine bleeding. It is commonly

326

performed to alleviate symptoms of conditions such as uterine fibroids and adenomyosis.

- **Myomectomy:** A myomectomy is a surgical procedure performed to remove uterine fibroids while preserving the uterus. Gynecologists can perform myomectomies using minimally invasive techniques such as laparoscopy or robotic-assisted surgery, providing a less invasive alternative to open abdominal surgery.

- **Pelvic Organ Prolapse Repair:** Gynecologists use minimally invasive techniques to repair pelvic organ prolapse, a condition in which the pelvic organs, such as the bladder, uterus, or rectum, descend into the vaginal canal. These procedures aim to restore pelvic organ support, alleviate symptoms, and improve quality of life.

Medical terms associated with gynecology facilitate effective communication, ensuring women get the health care they need. These complex terms also empower other health care professionals to support gynecologists who provide these services to patients.

As we wrap up Book 2 in this series, it's important to look back on what we've learned. So far, we've covered the structure of medical terms and given you the tools to decipher unfamiliar words yourself. We've also discussed how each specialized field of medicine uses specific terminology to discuss disorders, treatments, and subjects unique to that discipline.

In Book 3, we'll take this information a bit further and explain how how medical terms affect medical billing and coding specialists. You'll also find a glossary and other helpful resources that will give you the skills and confidence to tackle this challenging, rewarding career.

Chapter 8: An Introduction to Medical Coding

Welcome to the intriguing world of medical coding! In this chapter, we embark on a journey to unravel the mysteries of this vital component of the healthcare industry.

Medical coding involves the translation of medical diagnoses, procedures, and services into standardized codes that are recognized and understood by insurance companies, reimbursement systems, and healthcare professionals. By accurately assigning these codes, medical coders play a pivotal role in ensuring proper billing, claims submission, and reimbursement for healthcare services. So, let's dive into the depths of medical coding and discover the power of these codes, starting with an overview of their role in healthcare.

The Role of Medical Billing in Healthcare:

Medical coding bridges the complex world of medical documentation and administrative processes like billing, claims submission, and reimbursement. Medical coders create a standardized language that enables accurate and efficient communication among healthcare providers, insurance companies, and regulatory bodies by assigning specific codes to diagnoses, procedures, and services. These codes also provide crucial information for healthcare analytics, research, and decision-making.

Additionally, accurate coding ensures proper reimbursement for healthcare services, supports billing compliance, and helps prevent fraud and abuse. Without medical coding, the intricacies of healthcare documentation would remain incoherent, impeding effective healthcare management and hindering the ability to track and understand health trends.

Overview of Revenue Cycle Management

Revenue cycle management is the lifeblood of healthcare organizations. It encompasses a series of steps that healthcare providers follow to capture revenue for the services they render. From patient registration to charge capture, coding, claims submission, and reimbursement, each stage plays a vital role in maintaining the financial well-being of healthcare organizations.

Responsibilities of Billing Coders:

Billing coders are the superheroes of medical billing. They have the unique ability to translate complex medical documentation into a language that insurance companies and reimbursement systems understand. Their responsibilities include medical coding, charge entry, claims review, and denial management. Accurate and efficient coding ensures that healthcare providers receive the appropriate reimbursement for their services.

Basic Medical Billing Terms and Concepts

Anyone interested in medical billing and coding needs to understand complex and concepts. This section will explore the intricacies of healthcare insurance, medical documentation, coding, claims submission, and reimbursement methodologies.

After reading this section, you'll have a solid foundation in medical billing and be better equipped to navigate the ever-evolving landscape of healthcare finance.

Healthcare Insurance Terminology:

Anyone working in insurance reimbursement should understand the terminology related to health insurance, which can be confusing. Below are some common insurance-related terminology medical coders need to know:

Premiums: Regular payments individuals make to maintain their insurance coverage. These payments vary depending on factors such as age, location, and coverage type.

Deductibles: Predetermined amounts individuals must pay out of pocket before insurance coverage takes effect. This serves as a way to share the cost of healthcare services between the individual and the insurance provider. Once the deductible is met, individuals may be responsible for copayments and coinsurance.

Copayments: Fixed amounts that individuals must pay for specific services, such as doctor visits or prescription medications. For instance, a policy might require patients to pay $25 every time they visit the doctor.

Coinsurance: Unlike copayments, coinsurance represents a percentage of the cost of services that individuals are responsible for paying after meeting their deductible. In addition to the copayment, a patient's policy may require them to pay 10% of the total cost of treatment.

Medical Documentation and Coding:

Accurate and detailed medical documentation is the foundation for effective medical coding and billing. Healthcare providers document diagnoses, procedures, and services provided to patients. Medical coders then translate this documentation into standardized codes using coding systems such as ICD-10-CM (International Classification of Diseases, 10th Revision, Clinical Modification) for diagnoses and CPT (Current Procedural Terminology) for procedures.

Proper coding ensures that the correct information is communicated to insurance companies for claim submission and reimbursement. Medical coders must have a thorough understanding of coding guidelines, conventions, and documentation requirements to assign the appropriate codes accurately.

Claims Submission and Reimbursement:

Once the coding process is complete, medical coders submit the claim to the insurer. A claim is a request for reimbursement sent to insurance companies or other third-party payers. It includes all the necessary information, such as patient demographics, diagnosis codes, procedure codes, and charges.

Claims must be submitted accurately and in a timely manner to ensure proper reimbursement. The reimbursement process varies depending on the insurance plan and the reimbursement methodology. Fee-for-service is a common reimbursement model where healthcare providers are paid a predetermined fee for each service rendered.

Other reimbursement models include bundled payments, where a single payment covers multiple services related to a specific condition or procedure, and value-based reimbursement, where providers are reimbursed based on the quality of care they deliver.

Regulatory Compliance and Coding Audits:

Regulatory compliance is about following the rules and regulations that protect patient privacy and ensure ethical billing practices. You may have heard of the Health Insurance Portability and Accountability Act (HIPAA), which sets the standards for privacy and security in healthcare. Medical billing coders must meet the same privacy and accuracy standards as everyone else in the healthcare industry, so they're subject to regular audits.

Coding audits are checks on coding accuracy. They can be done internally or by external parties who specialize in auditing. The goal is to ensure that the coding is on point and aligned with the coding guidelines. Auditors review medical records, documentation, and coding practices to ensure everything is in order. They check if the right codes were assigned, modifiers were used correctly, and the documentation meets the requirements. Based on their findings, they provide feedback and suggestions for improvement.

This process helps protect patient privacy and ensures that sensitive information remains confidential and secure. Secondly, by complying with the regulations, healthcare organizations stay on the right side of the law and avoid penalties or legal issues. Audits also build trust with patients, insurance companies, and other stakeholders. When everyone knows that proper procedures are being followed and regulations are being met, it creates a sense of confidence and reliability.

Advanced Billing Concepts and Specialties

As a medical billing coder, understanding advanced concepts will elevate your expertise and expand your knowledge beyond the basics. This section will explore professional fee billing, hospital billing, and the nuances of third-party payers and managed care. By delving into these advanced billing concepts and specialties, you'll gain a deeper understanding of the complexities involved in medical coding and reimbursement.

Professional Fee Billing:
Professional fee billing is specific to physician practices and specialty clinics. It involves billing for professional services provided by physicians and other healthcare professionals.

Relative Value Units (RVUs) are used to determine the value of these services based on factors such as time, skill, and resources required. Fee schedules outline the reimbursement rates for specific services. The global period refers to the period during which additional services related to a previous procedure may be included in the initial reimbursement.

Hospital Billing:

Hospital billing is a unique area within medical billing. It encompasses billing for inpatient and outpatient services provided by hospitals. The UB-04 form is the standardized billing form used for hospital claims. Diagnosis-Related Groups (DRGs) are a classification system that groups similar diagnoses and procedures for reimbursement. The chargemaster is a comprehensive list of prices for all hospital services.

Third-Party Payers and Managed Care:

In the world of healthcare, third-party payers, such as insurance companies and government programs, play a significant role in reimbursement. Understanding their role and the intricacies of managed care is essential. Health Maintenance Organizations (HMOs) and Preferred Provider Organizations (PPOs) are managed care plans with specific reimbursement arrangements with healthcare providers. Exclusive Provider Organizations (EPOs) are another type of managed care plan that restricts coverage to specific providers.

Conclusion:

In this chapter, we navigated the complexities of medical billing terminology. Understanding these essential terms and concepts will empower you as a billing coder to accurately translate medical documentation into billing codes, facilitate claims submission, and ensure proper reimbursement. Remember, the field of medical billing is continually evolving, and staying updated with changes is crucial for success. In the next chapter, we'll take a closer look at some of the coding systems you'll use as a medical billing coder.

Medical billing coders use a variety of standards and codes to transfer medical information to insurance companies. In this chapter, we will explore the essential coding systems that serve as the backbone of medical documentation and reimbursement. These coding systems provide a standardized language for translating complex healthcare procedures, diagnoses, and services into universally recognized codes.

By understanding the intricacies of these coding systems, you'll gain a solid foundation for accurate and efficient coding practices. So, let's dive into the different coding systems you'll encounter in your career.

International Classification of Diseases (ICD)

The International Classification of Diseases (ICD) is a globally recognized coding system used for capturing diagnoses or medical conditions. It provides a comprehensive list of codes that represent various diseases, injuries, symptoms, and other health-related conditions. With ICD codes, medical coders can accurately code and classify a wide range of health conditions.

ICD-10-CM:

ICD-10-CM is the Clinical Modification of the International Classification of Diseases, 10th Revision. It is the coding system used for capturing diagnoses or medical conditions in healthcare settings. ICD-10-CM codes consist of alphanumeric characters and are designed to capture specific details about a patient's condition. These codes allow medical coders to document diagnoses with precision, facilitating accurate claims processing, epidemiological research, and statistical analysis.

ICD-10-PCS:

ICD-10-PCS is the Procedure Coding System of the International Classification of Diseases, 10th Revision. It is specifically used for coding medical procedures, particularly in hospital settings. ICD-10-PCS codes provide specific details about the procedures performed, including the body system involved, the approach used, and the device or substance involved. These alphanumeric codes allow for greater specificity and accuracy in coding procedures, ensuring appropriate reimbursement and precise documentation of medical services.

Current Procedural Terminology (CPT)

The Current Procedural Terminology (CPT) is a coding system developed by the American Medical Association (AMA) for describing medical procedures and services healthcare professionals provides. CPT codes serve as a standardized language for reporting and documenting medical services. Let's explore the different categories within the CPT coding system.

Category I Codes:

Category I codes are used for reporting commonly performed procedures and services. These codes cover a comprehensive range of medical specialties and enable precise reporting of services such as office visits, laboratory tests, surgeries, and consultations.

Each Category I code consists of five alphanumeric characters and includes a description of the procedure or service. Category I codes are regularly updated to keep pace with advancements in medical technology and evolving healthcare practices.

Category II Codes:

Category II codes are supplemental codes used for performance measurement and data collection. These codes allow for the standardized reporting of specific performance measures, such as patient history, patient education, and preventive services. While Category II codes are optional and not required for reimbursement, their inclusion provides valuable information for quality improvement, research purposes, and healthcare data analysis.

Category III Codes:

Category III codes are temporary codes used for emerging technologies and procedures. They facilitate the early identification and tracking of new and innovative medical procedures, services, and technologies. Category III codes are updated twice a year and are intended for temporary use until sufficient data is available to support the creation of permanent Category I codes.

These codes are critical in monitoring the effectiveness and safety of new procedures and technologies, ensuring accurate documentation, and facilitating appropriate reimbursement.

Healthcare Common Procedure Coding System (HCPCS)

The Healthcare Common Procedure Coding System (HCPCS) is a coding system used for reporting medical services and procedures not covered by CPT codes. It consists of two code levels: Level I and Level II codes. Let's explore the purpose and structure of HCPCS.

Level I Codes:

Level I codes in HCPCS are identical to CPT codes. These codes are used to report procedures and services performed by healthcare professionals. They cover a wide range of medical specialties and allow for accurate documentation and reimbursement of medical services. Level I codes follow the same structure and guidelines as CPT codes, ensuring consistency and interoperability across coding systems.

Level II Codes:

Level II codes in HCPCS are alphanumeric codes used to report medical supplies, equipment, non-physician services, and other items not covered by CPT codes. These codes provide a standardized method for reporting and billing various medical supplies, equipment, and services.

Level II codes are essential for accurate documentation, tracking healthcare utilization, ensuring appropriate reimbursement, and maintaining consistent reporting across healthcare settings.

Conclusion:

In this chapter, we explored the essential coding systems that drive the accurate documentation and reimbursement of medical services. The International Classification of Diseases (ICD), Current Procedural Terminology (CPT), and the Healthcare Common Procedure Coding System (HCPCS) form the core of medical coding, allowing for the standardized representation of diagnoses, procedures, and services.

ICD codes capture comprehensive details about diagnoses, while CPT codes enable precise reporting of procedures and services across medical specialties. HCPCS codes complete the coding landscape, covering medical supplies, equipment, non-physician services, and other items not captured by CPT codes.

Armed with this knowledge, you are well-equipped to navigate the dynamic world of medical coding systems and contribute to the accurate documentation and reimbursement of healthcare services.

In the next chapter, we'll leave the abstract theory behind and get into the practical application with concrete examples of medical billing and coding.

So far, we've learned a lot about the abstract concepts behind billing and coding, and developed an understanding of medical terminology. In this chapter, we'll explore the real-life implementation of medical coding and its crucial role in the reimbursement process. We'll take a look at practical examples, showcasing how medical coders translate clinical documentation into standardized codes across different coding systems.

By understanding the practical application of medical billing and coding, you will gain valuable insights into this essential healthcare discipline's day-to-day challenges and intricacies. So, let's dive into the practical world of medical coding and discover how medical terms are transformed into standardized codes.

Applying Medical Coding in Practice

Accurate and detailed documentation provides the necessary information for medical coders to assign appropriate codes that reflect the diagnoses, procedures, and services patients received. Medical coders carefully review patient records, including physician notes, laboratory results, and imaging reports, to extract the essential details needed for accurate code assignment.

Through comprehensive and precise documentation, medical coders ensure that healthcare services are adequately documented and that appropriate reimbursement is achieved.

Translating Medical Terms into Codes:

Medical coders use a variety of tools to translate medical terms into standardized codes. They utilize various coding systems, covered in the last chapter, to assign codes that accurately represent the diagnoses, procedures, and services provided to patients.

Let's explore practical examples of how medical terms are transformed into codes within different coding systems.

Practical Examples of Medical Coding

This section'll explore how medical coders translate clinical documentation into standardized codes. By delving into specific scenarios encountered in outpatient and inpatient settings, we'll examine common medical terms and their associated codes across different coding systems, such as ICD-10-CM and CPT.

- **Hypertension:** High blood pressure is prevalent in outpatient settings. It is coded using ICD-10-CM code I10 (Essential (primary) hypertension).

- **Diabetes mellitus is a chronic condition characterized by high blood sugar levels. The ICD-10-CM code for it** is E11.9 (Type 2 diabetes mellitus without complications).

- **Asthma is a** respiratory condition that causes wheezing, shortness of breath, and chest tightness. It is coded using ICD-10-CM code J45.909 (Unspecified asthma, uncomplicated).

- **Upper Gastrointestinal Endoscopy:** A procedure used to examine the lining of the upper digestive tract, including the esophagus, stomach, and duodenum. It is coded using CPT code 43239 (Upper gastrointestinal endoscopy including esophagus, stomach, and either the duodenum and/or jejunum as appropriate; diagnostic, with or without collection of specimen(s) by brushing or washing, with or without colon decompression (separate procedure)).

- **Appendectomy:** A surgical procedure to remove the appendix, often performed due to appendicitis. The corresponding CPT code for an appendectomy is 44950 (Appendectomy, routine).

- **Total Abdominal Hysterectomy:** This is a surgical procedure to remove the uterus through an incision in the abdomen. It is coded using CPT code 58150 (Total abdominal hysterectomy (corpus and cervix), with or without removal of tube(s), with or without removal of ovary(s)).

- **Acute Myocardial Infarction:** Also known as a heart attack, it occurs due to a blockage in the blood vessels supplying the heart muscle. The corresponding ICD-10-CM code is I21.9 (Acute myocardial infarction, unspecified).

- **Pneumonia is an** infection that inflames the air sacs in one or both lungs. The ICD-10-CM code for pneumonia is J18.9 (Pneumonia, unspecified organism).
- **Sepsis is a** life-threatening condition caused by the body's response to infection. It is coded using ICD-10-CM code A41.9 (Sepsis, unspecified organism).
- **Colonoscopy is a** procedure used to examine the inside of the colon and rectum. It is coded using CPT code 45378 (Colonoscopy, flexible; diagnostic, with or without collection of specimen(s) by brushing or washing, with or without colon decompression (separate procedure)).
- **Total Knee Replacement:** A surgical procedure to replace a damaged knee joint with an artificial one. The corresponding CPT code for total knee replacement is 27447 (Arthroplasty, knee, condyle, and plateau; medial and lateral compartments with or without patella resurfacing).
- **Cardiac Catheterization:** A procedure to diagnose and treat heart conditions using a catheter inserted into the blood vessels. It is coded using CPT code 93458 (Right heart catheterization including measurement(s) of oxygen saturation and cardiac output, when performed).

Cross-Referencing Across Coding Systems

Mapping ICD-10-CM to CPT:
Accurately linking ICD-10-CM and CPT codes is essential for appropriate reimbursement and claims processing. Medical coders ensure that the services provided align with the documented medical conditions by cross-referencing the diagnosis codes (ICD-10-CM) with the corresponding procedure codes (CPT).

This cross-referencing process guarantees that the procedures performed are directly related to the patient's diagnoses, supporting accurate reimbursement and claims adjudication.

HCPCS Codes in Practical Coding:

HCPCS Level II codes are crucial in reporting and billing medical supplies, equipment, non-physician services, and other items not covered by CPT codes. Medical coders utilize HCPCS codes to accurately document and report various healthcare items and services, such as durable medical equipment, ambulance services, prosthetics, orthotics, and supplies. By assigning the appropriate HCPCS codes, medical coders ensure that these additional services and items are accurately represented in the billing process.

- **Continuous Positive Airway Pressure (CPAP) Device:** HCPCS code E0601 represents CPAP devices used to treat obstructive sleep apnea. This code ensures accurate reporting and reimbursement for the rental or purchase of CPAP equipment and supplies.

- **Injection, Ketorolac Tromethamine:** HCPCS code J1885 is used to identify and bill for injections of Ketorolac Tromethamine, a nonsteroidal anti-inflammatory drug (NSAID) commonly administered for pain relief in various medical settings.

- **Walking Boot:** HCPCS code L4360 is assigned to walking boots used for immobilizing and supporting the foot and ankle following injuries or surgeries. This code helps in accurately documenting and billing for the provision of walking boots to patients.

- **Wheelchair, Manual, Pediatric:** HCPCS code E0181 is specific to manual wheelchairs designed for pediatric patients. This code ensures appropriate reimbursement for the rental or purchase of manual wheelchairs tailored to the unique needs of children.

- **Lancets:** HCPCS code A4253 is used to report and bill for lancets, which are small, sharp instruments used for pricking the skin to obtain blood samples for diagnostic testing, such as glucose monitoring in diabetic patients.

- **Infusion, Normal Saline Solution:** HCPCS code J7030 is used to identify and bill for the administration of normal saline solution intravenously or through other infusion methods. This code helps accurately document and reimburse for the provision of this common fluid therapy.

- **Durable Medical Equipment, Miscellaneous:** HCPCS code E1399 is a miscellaneous category code that covers various durable medical equipment (DME) items that do not have specific HCPCS codes assigned to them. It allows for the appropriate reporting and reimbursement of unique or less common DME supplies.

- **Non-Covered Item or Service:** HCPCS code A9270 is used to indicate that a specific item or service provided to a patient is not covered by the payer. It ensures proper documentation and billing for services or supplies that fall outside the scope of covered benefits.

- **Screening Papanicolaou (Pap) Smear:** HCPCS code Q0091 is used to report and bill for the collection of a screening Papanicolaou (Pap) smear, a test performed to detect cervical cancer or abnormalities in cervical cells. This code ensures accurate documentation and reimbursement for this preventive screening procedure.

- **Direct Referral for Patient Education:** HCPCS code G0154 is used to identify and bill for direct referrals to patient education programs, such as those related to diabetes management, nutrition counseling, or smoking cessation. This code helps in documenting and reimbursing the provision of these educational services.

These examples represent just a fraction of the many HCPCS codes utilized in medical billing and coding. The specificity and accuracy of HCPCS codes enable healthcare providers and insurers to document and process claims efficiently, ensuring appropriate reimbursement for the services and supplies provided to patients.

Conclusion:

Congratulations! You've reached the end of Book 3, and should have a strong understanding of medical billing and coding. Along with the practical application of medical billing and coding, we've also covered the basics of medical terminology, medical specializations, and anatomy.

We've also gained some insight into how medical coders translate clinical documentation into standardized codes across different coding systems. By understanding how medical coding is applied in practice, you can appreciate the significance of accurate documentation and proper code assignment.

The examples provided serve as valuable illustrations of the intricate process involved in converting medical terms into standardized codes. Armed with this knowledge, you are well-prepared to navigate the practical challenges of medical billing and coding, contributing to the accurate documentation, reimbursement, and overall efficiency of the healthcare system.

The following sections include resources designed to help you build the skills necessary for a successful career in medical billing and coding. Along with the enclosed flash cards, you can also work through the multiple-choice questions and exercises in the back of this book to apply the knowledge you've learned. We've also included a handy glossary of medical terms that can help you study.

Questions About Specializations, Diseases & Disorders

Answers to some of the questions below are included in this book. Others are included to encourage you to exercise the skills you've learned to figure out medical terms on your own.

1. **Which of the following specialists primarily treats disorders of the heart?**

   A. Neurologist

   B. Cardiologist

   C. Dermatologist

   D. Endocrinologist

2. **What is the main coding system used for diagnosing mental health conditions like depression and anxiety?**

   A. CPT

   B. ICD

   C. SNOMED

   D. HCPCS

3. **Which code would most likely be used for an annual flu vaccination?**

   A. E11.9

   B. J10.1

   C. Z23

   D. E66.01

4. **Which condition is classified as an autoimmune disorder?**

   A. Hypertension

   B. Diabetes Type 1

C. Tuberculosis

D. Osteoarthritis

5. **Which specialty deals with disorders of the nervous system, such as epilepsy?**

A. Pulmonology

B. Gastroenterology

C. Neurology

D. Endocrinology

6. **What type of specialist would treat skin conditions like eczema and psoriasis?**

A. Gastroenterologist

B. Cardiologist

C. Dermatologist

D. Oncologist

7. **What does the ICD-10 code 'E66.01' represent?**

A. Hypertension

B. Diabetes Type 2

C. Obesity due to excess calories

D. Influenza

8. **Which code category would you use to classify bone fractures?**

A. L codes

B. E codes

C. M codes

D. S codes

9. **Which type of diabetes is commonly diagnosed in children and requires insulin management?**

A. Type 1 Diabetes

B. Type 2 Diabetes

C. Gestational Diabetes

D. Prediabetes

10. **Which coding system is typically used for surgical procedures?**

A. ICD

B. CPT

C. LOINC

D. SNOMED

11. **What does the ICD code 'J45' represent?**

A. Hypertension

B. Asthma

C. Hyperlipidemia

D. Pneumonia

12. **Which of the following conditions is categorized as a chronic respiratory disorder?**

A. Influenza

B. Asthma

C. Bronchitis

D. Tuberculosis

13. **What condition would a rheumatologist most likely treat?**

A. Diabetes

B. Arthritis

C. Eczema

D. Depression

14. **In coding, which letter typically represents musculoskeletal conditions?**

A. M

B. N

C. R

D. T

15. **Which of the following is considered a genetic disorder?**

A. Hyperlipidemia

B. Cystic Fibrosis

C. Hepatitis

D. Hypertension

16. **The ICD-10 code 'F41.1' represents which mental health condition?**

A. Depression

B. Anxiety

C. Schizophrenia

D. Bipolar Disorder

17. **Which disease primarily affects the liver?**

A. Nephritis

B. Hepatitis

C. Meningitis

D. Gastritis

18. **What is the most common endocrine disorder treated by endocrinologists?**

A. Diabetes

B. Anemia

C. Osteoarthritis

D. Asthma

19. **Which type of cancer is often associated with HPV infection?**

A. Breast Cancer

B. Lung Cancer

C. Cervical Cancer

D. Prostate Cancer

20. **What is the primary focus of pulmonologists?**

A. Digestive system

B. Respiratory system

C. Nervous system

D. Cardiovascular system

21. **Which of the following codes would you use for a patient with chronic obstructive pulmonary disease (COPD)?**

A. K21.0

B. J44.9

C. N18.3

D. E11.65

22. **Who would be the primary specialist for treating Alzheimer's disease?**

A. Cardiologist

B. Gastroenterologist

C. Neurologist

D. Endocrinologist

23. **Which of the following conditions is commonly associated with obesity?**

A. Anemia

B. Sleep Apnea

C. Osteoporosis

D. Hypotension

24. **What is the most common cause of Type 2 diabetes?**

A. Genetic disorder

B. Autoimmune disease

C. Insulin resistance due to lifestyle factors

D. Viral infection

25. **Which code represents a diagnosis of hypertension?**

A. I10

B. E78.5

C. N40.1

D. J20.9

26. **A hematologist primarily treats disorders related to which of the following?**

A. Digestive system

B. Blood

C. Endocrine system

D. Respiratory system

27. **What is the ICD-10 code for Type 1 diabetes mellitus?**

A. E11

B. E10

C. E78

D. E66

28. **Which condition is characterized by progressive memory loss and cognitive decline?**

A. Parkinson's Disease

B. Alzheimer's Disease

C. Epilepsy

D. Multiple Sclerosis

29. **Which medical specialist is responsible for managing conditions related to hormones?**

A. Cardiologist

B. Dermatologist

C. Endocrinologist

D. Pulmonologist

30. **What does the code 'N18.4' represent in medical coding?**

A. Acute Kidney Injury

B. Stage 4 Chronic Kidney Disease

C. Hepatic Cirrhosis

D. Hyperlipidemia

31. **Which of the following diseases is commonly linked with vitamin D deficiency?**

A. Rickets

B. Anemia

C. Diabetes

D. Hypertension

32. **What is a common treatment goal for managing asthma in patients?**

A. Cure the disease

B. Control symptoms and prevent attacks

C. Increase lung capacity permanently

D. Eliminate the need for medication

33. **Which specialist is likely to treat gastrointestinal disorders like GERD and IBS?**

A. Endocrinologist

B. Gastroenterologist

C. Cardiologist

D. Neurologist

34. **The ICD-10 code 'C50' refers to cancer in which part of the body?**

A. Lung

B. Breast

C. Skin

D. Colon

35. **What is the primary focus of treatment for patients with congestive heart failure?**

A. Lowering blood sugar levels

B. Reducing fluid buildup and improving heart function

C. Increasing white blood cell count

D. Preventing blood clots

36. **Which condition is most likely treated by an immunologist?**

A. High blood pressure

B. Autoimmune disorders

C. Bone fractures

D. Type 2 diabetes

37. **Which specialist would most likely treat patients with hearing loss?**

A. Audiologist

B. Endocrinologist

C. Pulmonologist

D. Rheumatologist

38. **Which of the following is a chronic liver condition that can lead to cirrhosis?**

A. Asthma

B. Hepatitis C

C. Hypertension

D. Osteoporosis

39. **What does the ICD-10 code 'F32.0' represent?**

A. Generalized Anxiety Disorder

B. Mild Depression

C. Schizophrenia

D. Bipolar Disorder

40. **Which type of cancer is associated with abnormal growth of lymphatic cells?**

A. Leukemia

B. Lymphoma

C. Melanoma

D. Sarcoma

41. **Which specialist focuses on treating disorders of the urinary system?**

A. Cardiologist

B. Nephrologist

C. Urologist

D. Pulmonologist

42. **Which ICD-10 code is used for acute appendicitis?**

A. K35.80

B. I10

C. J44.9

D. E66.01

43. **Which of the following is an autoimmune disease affecting the thyroid?**

A. Graves' disease

B. COPD

C. Hypertension

D. Hepatitis

44. **What is the primary cause of anemia?**

A. Excessive vitamin intake

B. Insufficient red blood cells

C. High blood pressure

D. Blood clotting disorders

45. **Which ICD-10 code corresponds to chronic pain?**

A. R52

B. J45

C. I25.10

D. K52.9

46. **Which specialist would treat a patient with osteoporosis?**

A. Rheumatologist

B. Cardiologist

C. Gastroenterologist

D. Pulmonologist

47. **Which of the following conditions is categorized as a neurodegenerative disorder?**

A. Hypertension

B. Alzheimer's disease

C. Asthma

D. Gastritis

48. **What does the ICD-10 code E78.5 represent?**

A. Hypertension

B. Hyperlipidemia

C. Hypothyroidism

D. Chronic kidney disease

49. **Who is primarily responsible for treating skin cancer?**

A. Dermatologist

B. Oncologist

C. Endocrinologist

D. Rheumatologist

50. **Which of the following conditions affects the digestive system?**

A. Endometriosis

B. Diverticulitis

C. Myocardial infarction

D. Glaucoma

51. **Which specialist would manage disorders related to the pancreas, such as pancreatitis?**

A. Neurologist

B. Gastroenterologist

C. Pulmonologist

D. Dermatologist

52. **Which condition is characterized by high blood sugar levels due to insulin resistance?**

A. Type 1 Diabetes

B. Type 2 Diabetes

C. Addison's disease

D. Hyperthyroidism

53. **Which ICD-10 code is used for generalized anxiety disorder?**

A. F41.1

B. G40.1

C. J45.9

D. R51

54. **Which of the following is a condition primarily managed by a rheumatologist?**

A. Asthma

B. Osteoarthritis

C. Glaucoma

D. Peptic ulcer

55. **What type of disorder is COPD classified as?**

A. Cardiovascular

B. Endocrine

C. Respiratory

D. Gastrointestinal

56. **Which of the following codes is used to indicate chronic kidney disease, stage 3?**

A. N18.3

B. I10

C. E11.9

D. M19.9

57. **What specialist is responsible for diagnosing and treating vision problems?**

A. Nephrologist

B. Cardiologist

C. Ophthalmologist

D. Pulmonologist

58. **Which condition is commonly screened for with a mammogram?**

A. Cervical cancer

B. Breast cancer

C. Colon cancer

D. Prostate cancer

59. **What is the ICD-10 code for asthma?**

A. I10

B. F32

C. J45

D. E66.01

60. **Which ICD-10 code is typically used for patients with influenza?**

A. J10

B. M54.5

C. R11

D. F43.2

61. Which condition is commonly associated with high levels of cholesterol?

   - A) Hypertension

   - B) Hyperlipidemia

   - C) Anemia

   - D) Osteoporosis

62. What specialist would treat conditions like multiple sclerosis and Parkinson's disease?

   - A) Cardiologist

   - B) Neurologist

   - C) Pulmonologist

   - D) Dermatologist

63. Which ICD-10 code is used to indicate pneumonia?

   - A) J12.9

   - B) E11.9

   - C) I10

   - D) K21.0

64. Which of the following specialists primarily focuses on hormonal disorders?

   - A) Rheumatologist

   - B) Oncologist

   - C) Endocrinologist

- D) Nephrologist

65. What is the primary cause of osteoporosis?

  - A) Low bone density

  - B) High cholesterol

  - C) Liver dysfunction

  - D) Vitamin C deficiency

66. Which code would you use for an annual wellness visit without any abnormalities?

  - A) Z00.00

  - B) E66.01

  - C) N18.5

  - D) J10.1

67. What type of specialist would handle a case of severe asthma that's difficult to control?

  - A) Endocrinologist

  - B) Pulmonologist

  - C) Gastroenterologist

  - D) Cardiologist

68. Which condition is known as "adult-onset diabetes"?

  - A) Type 1 Diabetes

- B) Type 2 Diabetes

- C) Gestational Diabetes

- D) Prediabetes

69. The ICD-10 code 'K25.9' is used for which condition?

- A) Appendicitis

- B) Gastric ulcer

- C) Diabetes

- D) Asthma

70. Which specialty focuses on the treatment of diseases related to the kidneys?

- A) Nephrology

- B) Pulmonology

- C) Rheumatology

- D) Dermatology

71. Which ICD-10 code is used for an acute myocardial infarction (heart attack)?

- A) I21

- B) J45

- C) K35

- D) E10

72. Which of the following specialists treats cancer patients?

- A) Neurologist

- B) Oncologist

- C) Gastroenterologist

- D) Endocrinologist

73. What is the primary focus of a hematologist?

- A) Respiratory system

- B) Blood disorders

- C) Digestive system

- D) Skin conditions

74. Which ICD-10 code is used for insomnia?

- A) F51.9

- B) N18.9

- C) E66.9

- D) J10.1

75. Which specialist would most likely treat Crohn's disease?

- A) Gastroenterologist

- B) Cardiologist

- C) Dermatologist

- D) Pulmonologist

76. Which condition is characterized by inflammation of the joints?

- A) Osteoarthritis

- B) Pneumonia

- C) Hyperlipidemia

- D) Hypothyroidism

77. The ICD-10 code 'F33' is used to diagnose which condition?

- A) Schizophrenia

- B) Major depressive disorder, recurrent

- C) Bipolar disorder

- D) Generalized anxiety disorder

78. Which of the following is a common symptom of anemia?

- A) High blood pressure

- B) Fatigue

- C) Joint pain

- D) Skin rash

79. Which specialist would manage hormonal imbalances in adolescents with growth issues?

- A) Cardiologist

- B) Endocrinologist

- C) Pulmonologist

- D) Rheumatologist

80. Which condition is commonly associated with the ICD-10 code 'J20.9'?

   - A) Bronchitis, unspecified

   - B) Hypertension

   - C) Chronic kidney disease

   - D) Depression

81. Which ICD-10 code is used to indicate chronic sinusitis?

   - A) J32.9

   - B) I10

   - C) K21.0

   - D) E11

82. What is the primary role of a nephrologist?

   - A) Treat digestive disorders

   - B) Treat kidney diseases

   - C) Treat skin conditions

   - D) Treat lung conditions

83. Which condition is commonly associated with joint pain and stiffness, often treated by a rheumatologist?

   - A) Osteoarthritis

   - B) Hyperlipidemia

   - C) Pneumonia

- D) Diabetes

84. Which ICD-10 code is used for major depressive disorder, single episode?

  - A) F32.9

  - B) F41.1

  - C) E66.01

  - D) J10.9

85. Which specialist primarily focuses on treating blood cancers, such as leukemia?

  - A) Hematologist

  - B) Gastroenterologist

  - C) Neurologist

  - D) Pulmonologist

86. The ICD-10 code 'N40.1' is used for which condition?

  - A) Hypertension

  - B) Benign prostatic hyperplasia

  - C) Diabetes

  - D) Asthma

87. What is the main focus of a gastroenterologist?

  - A) Nervous system

- B) Cardiovascular system

- C) Digestive system

- D) Respiratory system

88. Which condition is characterized by high blood sugar levels during pregnancy?

- A) Type 1 Diabetes

- B) Gestational Diabetes

- C) Type 2 Diabetes

- D) Hyperlipidemia

89. Which ICD-10 code represents chronic obstructive asthma?

- A) J45.9

- B) J44.9

- C) E10

- D) I20

90. Which condition is most commonly associated with iron deficiency?

- A) Anemia

- B) Osteoarthritis

- C) Hypertension

- D) Hypothyroidism

91. Which specialist would treat a patient with chronic liver disease?

- A) Nephrologist

- B) Hepatologist

- C) Endocrinologist

- D) Cardiologist

92. Which ICD-10 code is used for an acute upper respiratory infection?

  - A) J06.9

  - B) I10

  - C) K21.9

  - D) E11.9

93. Which type of diabetes often occurs during pregnancy and typically resolves after childbirth?

  - A) Type 1 Diabetes

  - B) Type 2 Diabetes

  - C) Gestational Diabetes

  - D) Prediabetes

94. Which specialist would treat a patient with severe allergies and asthma?

  - A) Pulmonologist

  - B) Immunologist

  - C) Gastroenterologist

  - D) Nephrologist

95. The ICD-10 code 'K52.9' is used for which condition?

   - A) Gastroenteritis and colitis, unspecified

   - B) Hypertension

   - C) Diabetes

   - D) Asthma

96. What is the focus of an oncologist?

   - A) Heart diseases

   - B) Cancer treatment

   - C) Skin disorders

   - D) Endocrine disorders

97. Which condition is commonly screened for with a colonoscopy?

   - A) Colon cancer

   - B) Prostate cancer

   - C) Breast cancer

   - D) Lung cancer

98. Which ICD-10 code is used to indicate chest pain, unspecified?

   - A) R07.9

   - B) J45

   - C) E78.5

   - D) I10

99. Which specialist would most likely treat a patient with osteoporosis?

- A) Rheumatologist

- B) Cardiologist

- C) Neurologist

- D) Dermatologist

100. Which condition is associated with difficulty breathing and is often managed by a pulmonologist?

- A) Chronic obstructive pulmonary disease (COPD)

- B) Osteoarthritis

- C) Hyperlipidemia

- D) Hypothyroidism

ANSWERS

1. **B) Cardiologist**

2. **B) ICD**

3. **C) Z23**

4. **B) Diabetes Type 1**

5. **C) Neurology**

6. **C) Dermatologist**

7. **C) Obesity due to excess calories**

8. **D) S codes**

9. **A) Type 1 Diabetes**

10. **B) CPT**

11. **B) Asthma**

12. **B) Asthma**

13. **B) Arthritis**

14. **A) M**

15. **B) Cystic Fibrosis**

16. **B) Anxiety**

17. **B) Hepatitis**

18. **A) Diabetes**

19. **C) Cervical Cancer**

20. **B) Respiratory system**

21. **B) J44.9**

22. **C) Neurologist**

23. **B) Sleep Apnea**

24. **C) Insulin resistance due to lifestyle factors**

25. **A) I10**

26. **B) Blood**

27. **B) E10**

28. **B) Alzheimer's Disease**

29. **C) Endocrinologist**

30. **B) Stage 4 Chronic Kidney Disease**

31. **A) Rickets**

32. **B) Control symptoms and prevent attacks**

33. **B) Gastroenterologist**

34. **B) Breast**

35. **B) Reducing fluid buildup and improving heart function**

36. **B) Autoimmune disorders**

37. **A) Audiologist**

38. **B) Hepatitis C**

39. **B) Mild Depression**

40. **B) Lymphoma**

41. **C) Urologist**

42. **A) K35.80**

43. **A) Graves' disease**

44. **B) Insufficient red blood cells**

45. **A) R52**

46. **A) Rheumatologist**

47. **B) Alzheimer's disease**

48. **B) Hyperlipidemia**

49. **A) Dermatologist**

50. **B) Diverticulitis**

51. **B) Gastroenterologist**

52. **B) Type 2 Diabetes**

53. **A) F41.1**

54. **B) Osteoarthritis**

55. **C) Respiratory**

56. **A) N18.3**

57. **C) Ophthalmologist**

58. **B) Breast cancer**

59. **C) J45**

60. **A) J10**

61. **B) Hyperlipidemia**

62. **B) Neurologist**

63. **A) J12.9**

64. **C) Endocrinologist**

65. **A) Low bone density**

66. **A) Z00.00**

67. **B) Pulmonologist**

68. **B) Type 2 Diabetes**

69. **B) Gastric ulcer**

70. **A) Nephrology**

71. **A) I21**

72. **B) Oncologist**

73. **B) Blood disorders**

74. **A) F51.9**

75. **A) Gastroenterologist**

76. **A) Osteoarthritis**

77. **B) Major depressive disorder, recurrent**

78. **B) Fatigue**

79. **B) Endocrinologist**

80. **A) Bronchitis, unspecified**

81. **A) J32.9**

82. **B) Treat kidney diseases**

83. **A) Osteoarthritis**

84. A) F32.9

85. A) Hematologist

86. B) Benign prostatic hyperplasia

87. C) Digestive system

88. B) Gestational Diabetes

89. A) J45.9

90. A) Anemia

91. B) Hepatologist

92. A) J06.9

93. C) Gestational Diabetes

94. B) Immunologist

95. A) Gastroenteritis and colitis, unspecified

96. B) Cancer treatment

97. A) Colon cancer

98. A) R07.9

99. A) Rheumatologist

100. A) Chronic obstructive pulmonary disease (COPD)

Case Studies Using Real-World Examples

The internet offers a variety of free online databases of both CPT and ICD codes. Using what you've learned so far, combined with these resources and information from the previous book, *Medical Billing and Coding for Beginners,* try to find the answers to the scenarios below:

Exercise 1: Case Study: Patient A recently underwent a colonoscopy procedure. The physician performed a diagnostic colonoscopy with biopsy. The patient has private insurance, and the insurance company requires the use of CPT and ICD-10-CM codes. The physician's fee for the procedure is $1,200, and the allowable charge set by the insurance company is $900.

Exercise:

1. Determine the appropriate CPT code for the diagnostic colonoscopy with biopsy.

2. Assign the corresponding ICD-10-CM code for the reason of the procedure.

3. Calculate the patient's copayment if their insurance plan has a 20% coinsurance.

4. Calculate the amount the insurance company will reimburse the provider for the procedure.

Exercise 2: Case Study: Patient B visited an orthopedic specialist for a fracture of the left wrist. The physician performed an open reduction and internal fixation (ORIF) procedure. The patient has Medicare as their primary insurance. The physician's fee for the procedure is $2,500, and the Medicare fee schedule sets the allowable charge at $2,000.

Exercise:

1. Determine the appropriate CPT code for the ORIF procedure.

2. Assign the corresponding ICD-10-CM code for the left wrist fracture.

373

3. Calculate the Medicare payment based on the fee schedule and the Medicare's reimbursement rate.

4. Determine if the patient is responsible for any coinsurance or deductible.

Exercise 3: Case Study: Patient C visited a dermatologist for the removal of multiple benign skin lesions using cryosurgery. The physician performed cryosurgery on five lesions. The patient has a high-deductible health plan (HDHP). The physician's fee for each lesion removal is $200.

Exercise:

1. Determine the appropriate CPT code(s) for the cryosurgery procedure on multiple benign skin lesions.

2. Assign the corresponding ICD-10-CM code(s) for the skin lesions.

3. Calculate the total fee for the five lesion removals.

4. Determine the patient's responsibility based on their HDHP deductible.

Exercise 4: Case Study: Patient D visited an internist for a routine office visit. The physician provided a comprehensive examination and management of a chronic condition. The patient has Medicaid as their primary insurance. The physician's fee for the visit is $150.

Exercise:

1. Determine the appropriate CPT code for the comprehensive office visit.

2. Assign the corresponding ICD-10-CM code for the chronic condition.

3. Calculate the Medicaid reimbursement based on the fee schedule and the Medicaid's reimbursement rate.

4. Determine if the patient is responsible for any copayment.

374

Exercise 5: Case Study: Patient E underwent a laparoscopic cholecystectomy for the removal of the gallbladder. The surgeon performed the procedure using a laparoscope and multiple incisions. The patient has commercial insurance. The surgeon's fee for the procedure is $4,500, and the allowable charge set by the insurance company is $3,800.

Exercise:

1. Determine the appropriate CPT code for the laparoscopic cholecystectomy procedure.

2. Assign the corresponding ICD-10-CM code for the reason of the procedure.

3. Calculate the patient's coinsurance if their insurance plan has a 15% coinsurance.

4. Calculate the amount the insurance company will reimburse the provider for the procedure.

A

Abdomen: The abdomen refers to the area of the body between the chest and the pelvis. It contains various organs, including the stomach, liver, gallbladder, spleen, kidneys, and intestines. The abdomen is protected by the abdominal muscles and is a crucial region for digestion and nutrient absorption.

Adrenal glands: The adrenal glands are small, triangular-shaped glands located on top of the kidneys. These glands are responsible for producing essential hormones that play a vital role in regulating various bodily functions. The adrenal glands produce hormones such as cortisol, which helps regulate metabolism and stress response, and aldosterone, which helps regulate blood pressure and electrolyte balance.

Allergy: An allergy is an abnormal reaction of the immune system to a substance known as an allergen. Common allergens include pollen, dust mites, certain foods, and animal dander. When a person with allergies comes into contact with an allergen, their immune system reacts by releasing histamine and other chemicals, leading to symptoms such as sneezing, itching, nasal congestion, and watery eyes.

Anemia: Anemia is a condition characterized by a deficiency of red blood cells or hemoglobin in the blood. Red blood cells and hemoglobin are responsible for carrying oxygen throughout the body. When there is a shortage of these components, the body may not receive enough oxygen, leading to symptoms such as fatigue, weakness, pale skin, and shortness of breath. Anemia can be caused by various factors, including nutritional deficiencies, chronic diseases, and inherited conditions.

B

Biopsy: A biopsy is a medical procedure in which a small sample of tissue or cells is removed from the body for examination under a microscope. It is commonly performed to determine the presence of abnormal cells or to diagnose various conditions, including cancer. There are different types of biopsies, such as needle biopsy, incisional biopsy, and excisional biopsy, depending on the area of the body being examined and the nature of the suspected condition.

C

Cardiology: Cardiology is the medical specialty that focuses on the diagnosis and treatment of diseases and conditions related to the heart and blood vessels. Cardiologists are specialized physicians who are trained to diagnose and manage various heart conditions, such as coronary artery disease, heart failure, arrhythmias, and valvular heart disease. They use a combination of physical examinations, diagnostic tests, and medical interventions to provide comprehensive care for patients with cardiovascular problems.

CT scan (Computed Tomography): A CT scan, also known as a computed tomography scan, is a diagnostic imaging technique that uses X-rays and computer processing to create detailed cross-sectional images of the body. It provides a more detailed view of the internal organs, bones, and tissues compared to traditional X-rays. CT scans are commonly used to diagnose and monitor conditions such as tumors, fractures, infections, and internal injuries.

D

Dermatology: Dermatology is the medical specialty that deals with the diagnosis and treatment of disorders affecting the skin, hair, and nails. Dermatologists are physicians who specialize in managing various skin conditions, including acne, dermatitis, psoriasis, eczema, skin infections, and skin cancer. They perform skin examinations, prescribe medications, and may perform procedures such as biopsies, cryotherapy, and laser treatments to address skin concerns.

Diabetes: Diabetes is a chronic condition characterized by high levels of blood sugar (glucose). It occurs when the body either does not produce enough insulin or does not effectively use the insulin it produces. Insulin is a hormone that helps regulate blood sugar levels. There are different types of diabetes, including type 1 diabetes, type 2 diabetes, and gestational diabetes. Diabetes requires careful management, including blood sugar monitoring, medication or insulin therapy, dietary adjustments, and regular physical activity.

Diagnostic imaging: Diagnostic imaging refers to various techniques used to visualize the internal structures of the body for diagnostic purposes. It includes imaging modalities such as X-rays, CT scans, magnetic resonance imaging (MRI), ultrasound, and nuclear medicine scans. These imaging techniques provide valuable information to healthcare professionals in diagnosing and monitoring various conditions, allowing for timely and accurate treatment decisions.

E

Echocardiogram: An echocardiogram is a non-invasive diagnostic test that uses ultrasound waves to create images of the heart's structure and assess its function. It provides detailed information about the heart's chambers, valves, and blood flow patterns. Echocardiograms are commonly used to evaluate heart conditions, such as heart valve abnormalities, heart muscle function, and congenital heart defects.

Endocrinology: Endocrinology is the medical specialty concerned with the study of hormones and their related disorders. Endocrinologists diagnose and treat conditions related to hormone imbalances, such as diabetes, thyroid diseases, adrenal disorders, and reproductive hormone disorders. They work closely with patients to manage hormone-related conditions through medications, hormone replacement therapies, and lifestyle modifications.

ENT (Ear, Nose, and Throat): ENT, or otolaryngology, is the medical specialty that focuses on the diagnosis and treatment of disorders affecting the ear, nose, throat, and related structures. ENT specialists, also known as otolaryngologists, manage conditions such as ear infections, sinusitis, tonsillitis, voice disorders, hearing loss, and head and neck cancers. They perform examinations, provide medical treatments, and may perform surgeries to address specific ear, nose, and throat conditions.

Epilepsy: Epilepsy is a neurological disorder characterized by recurrent seizures caused by abnormal electrical activity in the brain. Seizures can vary in type and severity, ranging from momentary loss of awareness to convulsions. Epilepsy can be managed with antiepileptic medications, lifestyle modifications, and, in some cases, surgical interventions.

G

Gastroenterology: Gastroenterology is the medical specialty focused on the diagnosis and treatment of disorders affecting the digestive system. Gastroenterologists diagnose and manage conditions related to the esophagus, stomach, intestines, liver, pancreas, and gallbladder. They address issues such as gastroesophageal reflux disease (GERD), peptic ulcers, inflammatory bowel disease (IBD), liver diseases, and gastrointestinal cancers. Gastroenterologists may perform endoscopic procedures, such as colonoscopies and upper endoscopies, to diagnose and treat gastrointestinal conditions.

H

Hematology: Hematology is the branch of medicine dealing with the study of blood and blood disorders. Hematologists specialize in the diagnosis and treatment of conditions such as anemia, bleeding disorders, clotting disorders, leukemia, lymphoma, and various other blood-related disorders. They may perform blood tests, bone marrow examinations, and administer treatments like blood transfusions, chemotherapy, or stem cell transplantation.

Hypertension: Hypertension, commonly known as high blood pressure, is a medical condition characterized by elevated blood pressure levels. It is a significant risk factor for cardiovascular diseases, such as heart attacks and strokes. Hypertension can be managed through lifestyle modifications, including a healthy diet, regular exercise, stress management, and, in some cases, medication.

I

Immunology: Immunology is the branch of medicine that studies the immune system and its disorders. Immunologists investigate the body's immune response to infections, allergies, autoimmune diseases, and immunodeficiencies. They work to understand the mechanisms of immune reactions, develop therapies to modulate immune responses, and improve vaccine development.

Infectious disease: Infectious disease is a medical specialty focused on the diagnosis, treatment, and prevention of infections caused by microorganisms such as bacteria, viruses, fungi, and parasites. Infectious disease specialists play a crucial role in managing various infectious conditions, including respiratory infections, sexually transmitted infections, hepatitis, HIV/AIDS, and emerging infectious diseases. They employ a combination of diagnostic tests, antimicrobial medications, and infection control measures to effectively treat and prevent the spread of infectious diseases.

Infectious mononucleosis: Infectious mononucleosis, often called mono or the "kissing disease," is a viral infection caused by the Epstein-Barr virus (EBV). It is typically transmitted through saliva, hence its nickname. Symptoms include fatigue, sore throat, swollen lymph nodes, and fever. Treatment focuses on managing symptoms and allowing the body's immune system to fight off the infection.

J

Jaundice: Jaundice is a condition characterized by yellowing of the skin and whites of the eyes due to a buildup of bilirubin, a yellow pigment produced when red blood cells break down. It can be a symptom of liver disease, such as hepatitis or cirrhosis, or other medical conditions affecting the liver or bile ducts. Treatment depends on the underlying cause of the jaundice.

Joint replacement: Joint replacement, also known as arthroplasty, is a surgical procedure in which a damaged joint is removed and replaced with an artificial joint (prosthesis). It is commonly performed in individuals with severe joint pain or impaired mobility caused by conditions like osteoarthritis, rheumatoid arthritis, or joint trauma. Joint replacement surgeries most commonly involve the hip, knee, and shoulder joints.

K

Kidney stones: Kidney stones are hard deposits that form in the kidneys from substances in the urine. They can vary in size and shape and may cause severe pain as they pass through the urinary tract. Risk factors for kidney stones include dehydration, certain medical conditions, and a diet high in sodium or oxalate. Treatment options range from pain management and increased fluid intake to surgical removal of larger stones.

Kinesiology: Kinesiology is the study of human movement, particularly the mechanics and physiology of body movement. It applies scientific principles to assess and enhance physical performance, prevent injuries, and promote overall well-being. Kinesiologists often work with athletes, individuals recovering from injuries, and those seeking to improve their physical fitness through exercise and movement analysis.

L

Laparoscopy: Laparoscopy is a minimally invasive surgical technique that allows a surgeon to access and visualize the inside of the abdomen or pelvis using a small camera called a laparoscope. It is commonly used for diagnostic purposes or to perform surgical procedures such as gallbladder removal, appendectomy, or tubal ligation. Laparoscopy offers benefits such as smaller incisions, reduced scarring, and faster recovery compared to traditional open surgeries.

Lymph nodes: Lymph nodes are small, bean-shaped structures found throughout the body as part of the lymphatic system. They act as filters, trapping harmful substances and producing immune cells to fight infections. Swollen or enlarged lymph nodes can indicate an underlying infection or other medical condition. Lymph nodes are an important part of the body's immune response.

M

Magnetic resonance imaging (MRI): Magnetic resonance imaging (MRI) is a diagnostic imaging technique that uses a powerful magnetic field and radio waves to create detailed images of the body's internal structures. MRI provides excellent visualization of soft tissues, organs, and the brain, making it useful for detecting abnormalities, diagnosing diseases, and monitoring treatment progress. Unlike X-rays and CT scans, MRI does not use ionizing radiation.

Mammogram: A mammogram is a low-dose X-ray examination of the breasts used to detect and diagnose breast abnormalities, including tumors or cysts. Mammography plays a crucial role in breast cancer screening and early detection. Regular mammograms are recommended for women as they age or if they have a higher risk of breast cancer due to family history or other factors.

Microbiology: Microbiology is the study of microorganisms, including bacteria, viruses, fungi, and parasites. Microbiologists examine these organisms to understand their structure, function, and role in causing infectious diseases. They play a vital role in identifying pathogens, developing diagnostic tests, and researching treatments and preventive measures.

Migraine: A migraine is a recurring headache disorder characterized by moderate to severe throbbing pain, often accompanied by other symptoms such as nausea, vomiting, and sensitivity to light and sound. Migraines can be debilitating and significantly affect a person's quality of life. Treatment options range from lifestyle modifications and medications to manage and prevent migraines.

Multiple sclerosis (MS): Multiple sclerosis is a chronic neurological disease that affects the central nervous system, including the brain and spinal cord. It occurs when the immune system mistakenly attacks the protective covering of nerve fibers (myelin), leading to communication disruptions between the brain and other parts of the body. MS can cause a wide range of symptoms, including fatigue, balance problems, numbness, muscle weakness, and cognitive changes. Treatment aims to manage symptoms, slow disease progression, and improve quality of life.

N

Nephrology: Nephrology is the medical specialty focused on the diagnosis and treatment of kidney diseases and disorders. Nephrologists are specialized physicians who manage conditions such as kidney stones, chronic kidney disease, acute kidney injury, and kidney transplantation. They evaluate kidney function, monitor electrolyte and fluid balance, and develop treatment plans tailored to individual patients.

Neurology: Neurology is the medical specialty concerned with the diagnosis and treatment of diseases and conditions affecting the nervous system, including the brain, spinal cord, nerves, and muscles. Neurologists diagnose and manage a wide range of conditions such as stroke, epilepsy, multiple sclerosis, Parkinson's disease, and Alzheimer's disease. They use various diagnostic tests, including neuroimaging and neurological examinations, to assess and treat patients with neurological disorders.

O

Obstetrics: Obstetrics is the branch of medicine that focuses on the care of women during pregnancy, childbirth, and the postpartum period. Obstetricians provide prenatal care, monitor the health of the mother and fetus, and oversee the delivery process. They also manage any complications that may arise during pregnancy and ensure the well-being of both the mother and baby.

Oncology: Oncology is the medical specialty focused on the diagnosis and treatment of cancer. Oncologists specialize in managing different types of cancer, such as breast cancer, lung cancer, prostate cancer, and leukemia. They utilize various treatment modalities, including chemotherapy, radiation therapy, immunotherapy, and targeted therapies, to provide comprehensive cancer care.

Ophthalmology: Ophthalmology is the medical specialty concerned with the diagnosis and treatment of diseases and disorders of the eye and visual system. Ophthalmologists are specialized physicians who manage conditions such as cataracts, glaucoma, macular degeneration, and refractive errors. They perform eye examinations, prescribe corrective lenses, and perform surgical procedures, including cataract surgery and laser eye surgery.

P

Pulmonology: Pulmonology is the medical specialty focused on the diagnosis and treatment of diseases and conditions affecting the respiratory system, including the lungs and airways. Pulmonologists manage conditions such as asthma, chronic obstructive pulmonary disease (COPD), pneumonia, and lung cancer. They assess lung function, interpret diagnostic tests like pulmonary function tests and chest imaging, and develop treatment plans to improve respiratory health.

Psychiatry: Psychiatry is the medical specialty concerned with the diagnosis, treatment, and prevention of mental, emotional, and behavioral disorders. Psychiatrists evaluate patients for conditions such as depression, anxiety disorders, bipolar disorder, and schizophrenia. They provide counseling, prescribe medications, and may offer other therapies, such as cognitive-behavioral therapy, to address mental health concerns.

R

Radiology: Radiology is the medical specialty that focuses on the use of medical imaging techniques to diagnose and treat diseases. Radiologists interpret various imaging modalities, including X-rays, CT scans, MRI, ultrasound, and nuclear medicine scans, to aid in the diagnosis and management of various conditions. They work closely with other healthcare professionals to provide accurate and timely imaging interpretations.

Rheumatology: Rheumatology is the medical specialty focused on the diagnosis and treatment of diseases and conditions affecting the joints, muscles, and bones. Rheumatologists manage conditions such as arthritis, lupus, fibromyalgia, and osteoporosis. They assess patients' symptoms, perform physical examinations, order laboratory tests, and develop treatment plans to alleviate pain and improve function.

S

Scoliosis: Scoliosis is a medical condition characterized by an abnormal sideways curvature of the spine. It can develop during childhood or adolescence and may cause pain, postural abnormalities, and limited mobility. Treatment options for scoliosis range from observation and physical therapy to bracing or surgical intervention, depending on the severity and progression of the curvature.

Stroke: Stroke, also known as a cerebrovascular accident, occurs when blood flow to the brain is disrupted, leading to damage or death of brain cells. It can result from a blockage (ischemic stroke) or bleeding (hemorrhagic stroke) within the blood vessels of the brain. Prompt medical intervention is critical to minimize brain damage and improve outcomes. Treatment may involve medication, surgical procedures, or rehabilitation therapies.

T

Tonsillitis: Tonsillitis is an inflammation or infection of the tonsils, which are located at the back of the throat. It commonly presents with symptoms such as sore throat, swollen tonsils, difficulty swallowing, and fever. Tonsillitis can be caused by viral or bacterial infections. Treatment options include rest, fluids, pain relievers, and in some cases, antibiotic therapy or surgical removal of the tonsils (tonsillectomy).

Tuberculosis (TB): Tuberculosis is a contagious bacterial infection caused by Mycobacterium tuberculosis. It primarily affects the lungs but can also involve other organs. TB can be spread through the air when an infected person coughs or sneezes. Symptoms may include persistent cough, chest pain, fatigue, weight loss, and night sweats. Treatment involves a combination of antibiotics taken for several months to eradicate the infection.

U

Ulcer: An ulcer is an open sore or lesion that forms on the skin or mucous membranes. It can occur in various parts of the body, such as the stomach (gastric ulcer) or the skin (pressure ulcer). Ulcers can be caused by factors like infection, inflammation, poor blood circulation, or underlying medical conditions. Treatment aims to address the underlying cause, relieve symptoms, and promote healing.

Urology: Urology is the medical specialty focused on the diagnosis and treatment of conditions related to the urinary tract in both males and females, as well as the male reproductive system. Urologists manage conditions such as urinary tract infections, kidney stones, urinary incontinence, prostate disorders, and erectile dysfunction. They utilize diagnostic tests, medications, surgical procedures, and other interventions to address urological conditions.

V

Varicose veins: Varicose veins are swollen and twisted veins, usually in the legs, that result from damaged or weak valves within the veins. They can cause pain, discomfort, and visible bulging veins. Treatment options for varicose veins range from lifestyle modifications, compression stockings, and sclerotherapy (injection of a solution into the veins) to minimally invasive procedures or surgery for severe cases.

Viral gastroenteritis: Viral gastroenteritis, often referred to as stomach flu, is an inflammation of the stomach and intestines caused by a viral infection. It leads to symptoms such as nausea, vomiting, diarrhea, abdominal pain, and fever. The condition is usually self-limiting and resolves within a few days. Treatment involves supportive measures, such as staying hydrated and getting adequate rest.

W

Wound healing: Wound healing is the process by which the body repairs damaged tissues and restores skin integrity. It involves several stages, including inflammation, new tissue formation, and remodeling. Factors that can affect wound healing include the location and severity of the wound, underlying medical conditions, and individual factors. Proper wound care, including cleaning, dressing, and appropriate management, promotes optimal healing.

X

Xerostomia: Xerostomia, commonly known as dry mouth, is a condition characterized by reduced or absent saliva production. It can result from various factors, including medications, autoimmune diseases, radiation therapy, or salivary gland disorders. Xerostomia can lead to difficulties in speaking, swallowing, and an increased risk of dental problems. Treatment focuses on managing symptoms and addressing the underlying cause.

Y

Yellow fever: Yellow fever is a viral infection transmitted by infected mosquitoes, primarily in tropical and subtropical regions. It can cause flu-like symptoms, jaundice (yellowing of the skin and eyes), and potentially life-threatening complications. Yellow fever can be prevented through vaccination, and treatment involves supportive care to alleviate symptoms and manage complications.

Z

Zinc deficiency: Zinc deficiency is a nutritional deficiency that occurs when the body doesn't have enough zinc, an essential mineral involved in various bodily functions. Symptoms of zinc deficiency may include delayed growth and development, skin problems, impaired wound healing, hair loss, and compromised immune function. Zinc supplementation and dietary changes are the primary treatments for addressing zinc deficiency.

GET YOUR FREE BONUSES

Dear reader,

First and foremost, thank you for purchasing my book! Your support means the world to me, and I hope you find the information within valuable and helpful in your journey.

As a token of my appreciation, I have included some exclusive gifts that will greatly benefit you in your career.

Your Bonuses:

- **Audiobook**: The audiobook version of this book, Ideal for busy people, listen while commuting, during breaks, or at home to reinforce your knowledge and confidence to pass the certification exam.

- **Pharmacology Comprehensive ebook.** Expand your knowledge of pharmaceuticals and their interactions, gaining a deeper understanding of the medications and treatments used in healthcare.

- **Medical Prefixes and Suffixes ebook.** Explore the foundation of medical terminology, unraveling the meaning behind prefixes and suffixes commonly encountered in medical language.

- **Glossary of Terms ebook,** ensuring no term or definition is left unexplored. This valuable resource serves as a quick reference guide, facilitating your study and comprehension of medical terminology.

- **100 Digital and Printable Flashcards**: These digital and printable flashcards are an excellent tool to help you study and retain crucial information. They are designed to reinforce your knowledge, boost your confidence, and make learning enjoyable and convenient, whether you're on-the-go or at home. To use the flashcards I included a "README File" with the instructions.

I kindly ask you to take a moment to leave an honest review or rating of the book, it takes less than 30 seconds. Your feedback not only helps me improve my future work, but it also assists other readers in making informed decisions on their purchases. Please share your thoughts and experiences, as every review counts!

To access these bonuses, simply click on the link if you're using the ebook version, or scan the QR Code with your phone if you have the physical copy.

CLICK HERE FOR THE BONUSES

or
Scan this QR Code

Once again, thank you for your support, and I wish you the best of luck in your career. I believe these bonuses will provide you with the tools and knowledge to excel in this industry.

Medical Terminology and Anatomy

- **What does the prefix "hyper-" mean in medical terminology?**

A) Under, below

B) Excessive, above normal

C) Around, surrounding

D) Inside, within

- **The term "bradycardia" refers to:**

A) Fast heart rate

B) Slow heart rate

C) Inflammation of the heart

D) High blood pressure

- **Which suffix indicates "inflammation"?**

A) -ectomy

B) -osis

C) -itis

D) -pathy

- **In medical terminology, "nephro-" refers to which organ?**

A) Heart

B) Kidney

C) Liver

D) Lungs

- **The term "hematology" refers to the study of:**

A) Blood

B) Tissues

C) Cells

D) Bones

- **Which prefix means "half"?**

A) Mono-

B) Bi-

C) Semi-

D) Hyper-

- **The "myocardium" refers to:**

A) The outer layer of the skin

B) The muscular layer of the heart

C) The lining of the stomach

D) The membrane surrounding the lungs

- **Which of the following terms refers to low blood sugar?**

A) Hyperglycemia

B) Hypoglycemia

C) Hypotension

D) Hyperlipidemia

- **In anatomy, the "sagittal plane" divides the body into:**

A) Upper and lower halves

B) Front and back halves

C) Right and left halves

D) Diagonal sections

391

- **Which suffix is used to indicate "surgical removal"?**

A) -plasty

B) -ectomy

C) -tomy

D) -scopy

- **The term "osteoporosis" refers to:**

A) Inflammation of the bones

B) Excessive bone growth

C) Softening of the bones

D) Decrease in bone density

- **What does the prefix "tachy-" refer to?**

A) Slow

B) Fast

C) Above

D) Below

- **Which of the following refers to inflammation of the liver?**

A) Nephritis

B) Hepatitis

C) Gastritis

D) Arthritis

- **The "dermis" is part of which body system?**

A) Muscular system

B) Digestive system

C) Integumentary system

D) Respiratory system

- **The prefix "peri-" means:**

A) Within

B) Around

C) Between

D) Above

- **Which of the following terms refers to the study of tissues?**

A) Cytology

B) Hematology

C) Histology

D) Pathology

- **What does "cyanosis" indicate?**

A) Yellowing of the skin

B) Bluish discoloration due to lack of oxygen

C) Redness of the skin

D) Excessive sweating

- **Which body cavity contains the heart and lungs?**

A) Abdominal cavity

B) Cranial cavity

C) Thoracic cavity

D) Pelvic cavity

- **Which term refers to a condition of abnormal hardening?**

A) -sclerosis

B) -stasis

C) -lysis

D) -rrhea

- **Which part of the cell is responsible for energy production?**

A) Nucleus

B) Cytoplasm

C) Mitochondria

D) Cell membrane

- **What does the prefix "hypo-" mean in medical terminology?**

A) Above normal

B) Under, below normal

C) Around

D) Across

- **The term "arthralgia" refers to:**

A) Inflammation of the joints

B) Pain in the joints

C) Weakness in the joints

D) Excess fluid in the joints

- **Which of the following terms means "surgical repair"?**

A) -plasty

B) -stomy

C) -pathy

D) -lysis

- **The term "cephalalgia" refers to:**

A) Pain in the head

B) Pain in the chest

C) Pain in the abdomen

D) Pain in the back

- **The suffix "-cyte" refers to:**

A) A cell

B) A tissue

C) An organ

D) A muscle

- **Which of the following prefixes means "new"?**

A) Neo-

B) Retro-

C) Tachy-

D) Dys-

- **The "pericardium" refers to the:**

A) Muscular layer of the heart

B) Inner lining of the heart

C) Outer sac surrounding the heart

D) Blood vessels near the heart

- **Which term describes an abnormally low number of white blood cells?**

A) Leukopenia

B) Leukocytosis

C) Thrombocytosis

D) Polycythemia

- **The term "hepatomegaly" means:**

A) Inflammation of the liver

B) Abnormal enlargement of the liver

C) Cancer of the liver

D) Stone in the liver

- **Which plane divides the body into front and back sections?**

A) Sagittal plane

B) Frontal (coronal) plane

C) Transverse plane

D) Oblique plane

- **What is the term for pain in a muscle?**

A) Myalgia

B) Arthralgia

C) Myopathy

D) Ostealgia

- **Which prefix refers to "stomach"?**

A) Hepato-

B) Nephro-

C) Gastro-

D) Neuro-

- **Which term refers to the study of the skin and its diseases?**

A) Cytology

B) Dermatology

C) Pathology

D) Urology

• **The suffix "-emia" refers to a condition of the:**

A) Skin

B) Bones

C) Blood

D) Lungs

• **Which of the following means "difficult or painful digestion"?**

A) Dyspnea

B) Dysphagia

C) Dyspepsia

D) Dystrophy

• **Which of the following body systems is responsible for producing hormones?**

A) Nervous system

B) Endocrine system

C) Integumentary system

D) Muscular system

• **What does the term "thoracotomy" mean?**

A) Incision into the thoracic cavity

B) Removal of a lung

C) Inflammation of the chest wall

D) Imaging of the lungs

- **The term "adipose" refers to:**

A) Blood tissue

B) Bone tissue

C) Fat tissue

D) Muscle tissue

- **The term "cystectomy" refers to:**

A) Removal of the bladder

B) Removal of a cyst

C) Removal of the liver

D) Removal of a kidney

- **Which suffix means "to view or examine"?**

A) -scope

B) -graphy

C) -scopy

D) -gram

- **Which of the following terms means "abnormal softening"?**

A) -sclerosis

B) -malacia

C) -stasis

D) -algia

- **What does the prefix "contra-" mean?**

A) Against

B) Before

C) Around

D) Within

- **The term "cholecystectomy" refers to the surgical removal of the:**

A) Gallbladder

B) Liver

C) Kidney

D) Pancreas

- **What does the suffix "-megaly" mean?**

A) Pain

B) Enlargement

C) Tumor

D) Inflammation

- **Which term refers to an irregular heartbeat?**

A) Dysphagia

B) Arrhythmia

C) Aphasia

D) Aneurysm

- **Which of the following prefixes means "many" or "much"?**

A) Poly-

B) Hypo-

C) Dys-

D) Mono-

- **The term "nephrolithiasis" refers to the presence of:**

A) Fluid in the lungs

B) Stones in the kidney

C) Infection in the liver

D) Blood clots in the heart

- **What is the medical term for inflammation of the tonsils?**

A) Tonsillectomy

B) Tonsillitis

C) Tonsillopathy

D) Tonsilloscopy

- **Which term refers to the surgical removal of the appendix?**

A) Appendicitis

B) Appendectomy

C) Appendopathy

D) Appendotomy

- **The suffix "-pathy" refers to:**

A) Disease

B) Pain

C) Inflammation

D) Condition

- **Which of the following prefixes means "outside" or "outer"?**

A) Endo-

B) Ecto-

C) Intra-

D) Hypo-

- **Which medical term describes difficulty swallowing?**

A) Dysphasia

B) Dysplasia

C) Dysphagia

D) Dyspnea

- **Which of the following terms means "inflammation of the joints"?**

A) Arthritis

B) Arthroscopy

C) Arthralgia

D) Arthroplasty

- **Which term means "surgical creation of an opening"?**

A) -stomy

B) -otomy

C) -scopy

D) -pexy

- **What does the prefix "inter-" mean?**

A) Inside

B) Between

C) Above

D) Below

- **The term "cyanoderma" refers to:**

A) Redness of the skin

B) Blue discoloration of the skin

C) Yellowing of the skin

D) Hardening of the skin

- **Which body system does the "hepatic" refer to?**

A) Respiratory system

B) Urinary system

C) Digestive system

D) Muscular system

- **What does the term "osteomalacia" mean?**

A) Softening of the bone

B) Bone inflammation

C) Bone infection

D) Hardening of the bone

- **The term "meningitis" refers to inflammation of the:**

A) Muscles

B) Brain lining

C) Bones

D) Heart lining

- **Which of the following prefixes means "white"?**

A) Erythr-

B) Melano-

C) Leuko-

D) Xanth-

- **What does the prefix "endo-" mean in medical terminology?**

  A) Outside

  B) Within

  C) Above

  D) Below

- **The term "pneumonia" refers to:**

  A) Inflammation of the lungs

  B) Inflammation of the stomach

  C) Inflammation of the heart

  D) Inflammation of the kidneys

- **Which suffix indicates "study of"?**

  A) -logy

  B) -itis

  C) -ectomy

  D) -pathy

- **In medical terminology, "cardio-" refers to which organ?**

  A) Brain

  B) Heart

  C) Stomach

  D) Liver

- **The term "neurotransmitter" refers to a substance that:**

A) Transmits signals across the brain

B) Helps in digestion

C) Regulates blood pressure

D) Affects heart rate

- **Which prefix means "before"?**

A) Post-

B) Pre-

C) Intra-

D) Supra-

- **The term "dermatitis" refers to:**

A) Inflammation of the skin

B) Inflammation of the heart

C) Inflammation of the lungs

D) Inflammation of the brain

- **Which suffix indicates a condition or state?**

A) -osis

B) -ectomy

C) -scopy

D) -itis

- **What does the prefix "trans-" mean?**

A) Within

B) Across

C) Above

D) Below

- **The term "splenomegaly" refers to:**

A) Enlargement of the spleen

B) Inflammation of the spleen

C) Removal of the spleen

D) Infection of the spleen

- **What does the prefix "ab-" mean in medical terminology?**

A) Toward

B) Away from

C) Against

D) Above

- **The term "gastroenteritis" refers to:**

A) Inflammation of the liver

B) Inflammation of the stomach and intestines

C) Inflammation of the pancreas

D) Inflammation of the gallbladder

- **Which suffix means "condition of"?**

    A) -itis

    B) -osis

    C) -ectomy

    D) -plasty

- **In medical terminology, "osteo-" refers to which tissue?**

    A) Muscle

    B) Blood

    C) Bone

    D) Nerve

- **The term "hypertension" refers to:**

    A) Low blood pressure

    B) High blood pressure

    C) Normal blood pressure

    D) Fluctuating blood pressure

- **Which prefix means "through" or "across"?**

    A) Inter-

    B) Intra-

    C) Per-

    D) Sub-

- **The term "nephrectomy" refers to:**

A) Removal of the kidney

B) Removal of the bladder

C) Removal of a cyst

D) Removal of a tumor

- **Which suffix indicates "pain"?**

A) -itis

B) -algia

C) -ectomy

D) -osis

- **What does the prefix "ultra-" mean?**

A) Below

B) Above or beyond

C) Within

D) Outside

- **The term "cholelithiasis" refers to the presence of:**

A) Gallstones

B) Liver stones

C) Kidney stones

D) Blood clots

- **What does the prefix "dys-" mean in medical terminology?**

A) Normal

B) Difficult or painful

C) Good

D) Fast

- **The term "hyperlipidemia" refers to:**

A) Low levels of fat in the blood

B) High levels of fat in the blood

C) Normal levels of fat in the blood

D) Inflammation of the fat tissue

- **Which suffix indicates "enlargement"?**

A) -itis

B) -megaly

C) -ectomy

D) -algia

- **In medical terminology, "hemat-" refers to which substance?**

A) Tissue

B) Nerve

C) Blood

D) Bone

- **The term "colitis" refers to:**

  A) Inflammation of the colon

  B) Inflammation of the stomach

  C) Inflammation of the liver

  D) Inflammation of the pancreas

- **Which prefix means "against"?**

  A) Anti-

  B) Contra-

  C) Pre-

  D) Hyper-

- **The term "thrombocytopenia" refers to:**

  A) Low platelet count

  B) High platelet count

  C) Low red blood cell count

  D) High white blood cell count

- **Which suffix indicates "surgical creation of an opening"?**

  A) -stomy

  B) -tomy

  C) -scopy

  D) -ectomy

- **What does the prefix "circum-" mean?**

A) Across

B) Around

C) Between

D) Above

- **The term "asphyxia" refers to:**

A) Lack of oxygen

B) Excessive oxygen

C) Heart failure

D) Low blood pressure

- **What does the prefix "retro-" mean in medical terminology?**

A) Before

B) Behind or backward

C) Outside

D) Above

- **The term "pulmonary" refers to:**

A) Relating to the heart

B) Relating to the lungs

C) Relating to the stomach

D) Relating to the kidneys

- **Which suffix indicates "abnormal condition"?**

A) -ectomy

B) -itis

C) -osis

D) -plasty

- **In medical terminology, "cyto-" refers to which structure?**

A) Tissue

B) Cell

C) Organ

D) Bone

- **The term "febrile" refers to:**

A) Low temperature

B) High temperature

C) Normal temperature

D) Fluctuating temperature

- **Which prefix means "within" or "inside"?**

A) Ecto-

B) Endo-

C) Exo-

D) Inter-

- **The term "encephalitis" refers to:**

  A) Inflammation of the brain

  B) Inflammation of the liver

  C) Inflammation of the lungs

  D) Inflammation of the heart

- **Which suffix indicates "condition of the blood"?**

  A) -emia

  B) -osis

  C) -itis

  D) -pathy

- **What does the prefix "micro-" mean?**

  A) Large

  B) Small

  C) Many

  D) Fast

- **The term "anemia" refers to:**

  A) High red blood cell count

  B) Low red blood cell count

  C) Low white blood cell count

  D) High white blood cell count

ANSWERS

1. **B) Under, below normal**
2. **B) Pain in the joints**
3. **A) -plasty**
4. **A) Pain in the head**
5. **A) A cell**
6. **A) Neo-**
7. **C) Outer sac surrounding the heart**
8. **A) Leukopenia**
9. **B) Abnormal enlargement of the liver**
10. **B) Frontal (coronal) plane**
11. **A) Myalgia**
12. **C) Gastro-**
13. **B) Dermatology**
14. **C) Blood**
15. **C) Dyspepsia**
16. **B) Endocrine system**
17. **A) Incision into the thoracic cavity**
18. **C) Fat tissue**
19. **A) Removal of the bladder**
20. **C) -scopy**
21. **B) -malacia**
22. **A) Against**
23. **A) Gallbladder**

24. **B) Enlargement**

25. **B) Arrhythmia**

26. **A) Poly-**

27. **B) Stones in the kidney**

28. **B) Tonsillitis**

29. **B) Appendectomy**

30. **A) Disease**

31. **B) Ecto-**

32. **C) Dysphagia**

33. **A) Arthritis**

34. **A) -stomy**

35. **B) Between**

36. **B) Blue discoloration of the skin**

37. **C) Digestive system**

38. **A) Softening of the bone**

39. **B) Brain lining**

40. **C) Leuko-**

41. **B) Under, below normal**

42. **B) Pain in the joints**

43. **A) -plasty**

44. **A) Pain in the head**

45. **A) A cell**

46. **A) Neo-**

47. **C) Outer sac surrounding the heart**

48. **A) Leukopenia**

49. **B) Abnormal enlargement of the liver**

50. **B) Frontal (coronal) plane**

51. **A) Myalgia**

52. **C) Gastro-**

53. **B) Dermatology**

54. **C) Blood**

55. **C) Dyspepsia**

56. **B) Endocrine system**

57. **A) Incision into the thoracic cavity**

58. **C) Fat tissue**

59. **A) Removal of the bladder**

60. **C) -scopy**

61. B) Within

62. A) Inflammation of the lungs

63. A) -logy

64. B) Heart

65. A) Transmits signals across the brain

66. B) Pre-

67. A) Inflammation of the skin

68. A) -osis

69. B) Across

70. A) Enlargement of the spleen

71. B) Away from

415

72. B) Inflammation of the stomach and intestines

73. B) -osis

74. C) Bone

75. B) High blood pressure

76. C) Per-

77. A) Removal of the kidney

78. B) -algia

79. B) Above or beyond

80. A) Gallstones

81. B) Difficult or painful

82. B) High levels of fat in the blood

83. B) -megaly

84. C) Blood

85. A) Inflammation of the colon

86. A) Anti-

87. A) Low platelet count

88. A) -stomy

89. B) Around

90. A) Lack of oxygen

91. B) Behind or backward

92. B) Relating to the lungs

93. C) -osis

94. B) Cell

95. B) High temperature

96. B) Endo-

97. A) Inflammation of the brain

98. A) -emia

99. B) Small

100. B) Low red blood cell count

About Medical Billing and Coding

1. **Which coding system is primarily used to report diagnoses in the United States?**

A. CPT

B. ICD-10-CM

C. HCPCS Level II

D. SNOMED

2. **What does the CPT code set primarily cover?**

A. Diagnostic codes

B. Surgical procedures and medical services

C. Medical equipment

D. Patient demographics

3. **Which organization is responsible for maintaining the ICD-10-CM codes?**

A. American Medical Association (AMA)

B. Centers for Medicare & Medicaid Services (CMS)

C. World Health Organization (WHO)

D. American Health Information Management Association (AHIMA)

4. **What does the acronym HCPCS stand for?**

A. Healthcare Common Procedure Coding System

B. Health Coding and Procedure System

C. Health Coverage Procedure Coding System

D. Hospital Common Procedure Coding System

5. **Which of the following is a modifier in CPT coding that indicates a bilateral procedure?**

A. 50

B. 22

C. 25

D. 76

6. **What is the main purpose of medical billing?**

A. To diagnose patient conditions

B. To ensure healthcare providers are paid for services rendered

C. To maintain patient records

D. To assist in patient care management

7. **Which ICD-10-CM code category is used for external causes of injury?**

A. E codes

B. F codes

C. V codes

D. Z codes

8. **Which code set is used to classify equipment, supplies, and products not covered by CPT?**

A. ICD-10-CM

B. CPT

C. SNOMED CT

D. HCPCS Level II

9. **What is upcoding in medical billing?**

A. Billing for a higher level of service than was provided

B. Billing for a lower level of service than was provided

C. Billing the same service multiple times

D. Using an outdated code set

10. **What modifier would you use to indicate that a service provided was significantly more complex than usual?**

A. 25

B. 59

C. 22

D. 91

11. **Which of the following describes the purpose of CPT Category II codes?**

A. Experimental services and emerging technology

B. Medical procedures and services

C. Tracking performance measures

D. Durable medical equipment

12. **What is unbundling in medical coding?**

A. Combining codes to simplify billing

B. Using separate codes for procedures that should be billed together

C. Using a single code for multiple services

D. Billing for services that were not provided

13. **Which code in ICD-10-CM represents hypertension without complications?**

A. E11.9

B. I10

C. J45.9

D. R03.0

14. **In HCPCS Level II codes, what letter typically represents codes for durable medical equipment?**

A. J

B. K

C. L

D. D

15. **What does the "Z" code category in ICD-10-CM represent?**

A. External causes of injury

B. Infectious diseases

C. Factors influencing health status and contact with health services

D. Mental health disorders

16. **Which type of code would you use for a routine physical examination in ICD-10-CM?**

A. E code

B. Z code

C. T code

D. V code

17. **Which organization is primarily responsible for updating CPT codes?**

A. American Medical Association (AMA)

B. Centers for Medicare & Medicaid Services (CMS)

C. World Health Organization (WHO)

D. National Center for Health Statistics (NCHS)

18. **What is the purpose of a coding audit in healthcare?**

A. To train new coding specialists

B. To ensure accuracy and compliance with coding standards

C. To assist patients with billing inquiries

D. To update electronic health records

19. **Which of the following is an example of a place of service code used in medical billing?**

A. 21 - Inpatient Hospital

B. 25 - Emergency Room

C. 41 - Home

D. 50 - Ambulatory Surgery Center

20. **In medical coding, what is a "global period"?**

A. The time frame when all services related to a procedure are included in the original charge

B. The time frame for billing procedures

C. The period allowed for a patient to make payments

D. The duration a code remains valid in the coding system

21. **What does ICD-10-CM stand for?**

A. International Coding of Diseases, 10th Revision - Clinical Modifiers

B. International Classification of Diseases, 10th Revision - Clinical Modification

C. International Code for Diagnoses, 10th Revision - Clinical Modifiers

D. International Code for Doctors, 10th Revision - Classification Method

22. **What is the purpose of CPT Category III codes?**

A. For diagnostic procedures

B. For experimental and emerging technologies

C. For general medical services

D. For durable medical equipment

23. **In ICD-10-CM coding, which letter is not used in any codes?**

A. U

B. Y

C. W

D. Z

24. **What does the modifier "-99" indicate in CPT coding?**

A. Multiple modifiers are applied

B. A procedure is bilateral

C. The procedure is more complex than usual

D. A reduced service was provided

25. **Which of the following best describes "medical necessity"?**

A. Any service requested by the patient

B. A service that is covered by all insurance plans

C. A service that is necessary for the diagnosis or treatment of a patient's condition

D. A service that is elective or optional

26. **Which type of code would most likely be used for a patient with a fractured femur?**

A. M code

B. S code

C. E code

D. J code

27. **What is a common coding error related to sequencing in ICD-10-CM?**

A. Upcoding

B. Unbundling

C. Incorrect primary diagnosis order

D. Misusing modifiers

28. **What is the main purpose of modifiers in medical coding?**

A. To create new codes

B. To provide additional information about a procedure or service

C. To reduce the cost of a procedure

D. To increase the complexity of a procedure

29. **Which CPT modifier would indicate that a procedure was repeated?**

A. 25

B. 91

C. 76

D. 59

30. **What code category in ICD-10-CM is used for symptoms, signs, and abnormal clinical findings?**

A. A00-B99

B. E00-E89

C. R00-R99

D. S00-T88

31. **Which code is used for documenting preventive healthcare services?**

A. Z codes in ICD-10-CM

B. T codes in ICD-10-CM

C. L codes in ICD-10-CM

D. D codes in ICD-10-CM

32. **What is downcoding?**

A. Assigning a lower code than what was performed

B. Billing for multiple codes when one would suffice

C. Using outdated codes

D. Assigning a higher code than what was performed

33. **In medical billing, which of the following is a common denial reason?**

A. Duplicate claim

B. Correct modifier usage

C. Valid place of service code

D. Payment approved

34. **What code system is used for coding vaccines and injectable drugs?**

A. CPT

B. HCPCS Level II

C. ICD-10-CM

D. SNOMED CT

35. **What is the role of a claims adjuster in the medical billing process?**

A. To diagnose patients

B. To negotiate claim settlements with insurance companies

C. To review and approve or deny insurance claims

D. To set healthcare service prices

36. **Which coding system is used for hospital inpatient procedures in the U.S.?**

A. ICD-10-PCS

B. CPT

C. HCPCS Level II

D. ICD-10-CM

37. **What does "bundling" mean in medical coding?**

A. Combining two or more related codes into a single code

B. Using multiple codes for one procedure

C. Submitting duplicate claims

D. Coding for services not provided

38. **In ICD-10-CM, what does the "X" character represent in codes?**

A. Diagnosis unknown

B. Placeholder character

C. Increased specificity

D. Indicates an injury

39. **What code type is used for reporting physical therapy procedures?**

A. E codes

B. CPT codes

C. Z codes

D. T codes

40. **What type of code in HCPCS Level II is commonly used for ambulance services?**

A. G codes

B. A codes

C. K codes

D. L codes

41. **Which of the following is a common tool used by coders to ensure accurate code selection?**

A. Insurance policy

B. Coding manual

C. Patient chart

D. Healthcare bill

42. **Which CPT code category is used for E/M services?**

A. Category I

B. Category II

C. Category III

D. Category IV

43. **Which organization publishes the Current Procedural Terminology (CPT) codes?**

A. World Health Organization (WHO)

B. Centers for Disease Control and Prevention (CDC)

C. Centers for Medicare & Medicaid Services (CMS)

D. American Medical Association (AMA)

44. **Which modifier indicates that a service was performed on the right side of the body?**

A. -50

B. -RT

C. -LT

D. -51

45. **Which part of Medicare primarily covers inpatient hospital care?**

A. Part A

B. Part B

C. Part C

D. Part D

46. **What is the purpose of the superbill in medical billing?**

A. To record a patient's complete medical history

B. To track insurance payments

C. To document the services provided and their corresponding codes for billing

D. To schedule appointments

47. **Which of the following is an example of fraud in medical billing?**

A. Using an outdated code by accident

B. Billing for services not provided

C. Failing to code a service

D. Submitting a claim with a typo

48. **What does "payer" refer to in medical billing?**

A. The patient receiving treatment

B. The hospital administrator

C. The insurance company responsible for payment

D. The healthcare provider offering services

49. **Which of the following codes is used for anesthesia services?**

A. CPT codes 10021-69990

B. CPT codes 00100-01999

C. CPT codes 70010-79999

D. CPT codes 90010-99999

50. **What type of form is used to submit claims to Medicare and most other insurance payers?**

A. CMS-1500

B. UB-04

C. ICD-10 form

D. CPT-04

51. **What does the "-99" modifier indicate in medical coding?**

A. The procedure was reduced

B. Multiple procedures were performed

C. Multiple modifiers apply to the code

D. The service was provided outside of normal hours

52. **What is the term for the amount a patient is required to pay out of pocket before insurance covers the rest?**

A. Premium

B. Deductible

C. Co-payment

D. Coinsurance

53. **What is the primary function of ICD-10-PCS codes?**

A. To code inpatient procedures

B. To code outpatient visits

C. To code for billing only

D. To code for anesthesia services

54. **Which modifier indicates a professional service only, such as an interpretation of a diagnostic test?**

A. -26

B. -50

C. -TC

D. -51

55. **Which of the following is a reason for claim denial due to lack of medical necessity?**

A. Service was not documented

B. Service was coded incorrectly

C. Service was not justified by patient's diagnosis

D. Service was provided on the wrong date

56. **Which coding system is specifically used to code dental services?**

A. ICD-10-CM

B. CPT

C. HCPCS Level II

D. CDT

57. **Which of the following statements best describes the "allowed amount"?**

A. The total cost billed by the provider

B. The maximum amount an insurance company will pay for a service

C. The amount paid directly by the patient

D. The annual limit on patient's out-of-pocket expenses

58. **What does the term "assignment of benefits" mean in medical billing?**

A. The provider agrees to accept the insurance payment as full payment

B. The patient pays the entire bill upfront

C. The provider bills the patient directly instead of the insurance company

D. The provider accepts a lower payment for quicker processing

59. **Which type of code is used to report the administration of a flu shot?**

A. CPT

B. ICD-10-CM

C. HCPCS Level II

D. CDT

60. **In billing, what is "coinsurance"?**

A. A fixed amount paid by the patient for a service

B. The percentage of a service cost shared between patient and insurer

C. The full amount billed to the patient

D. The amount the insurance company pays directly to the provider

61. What is the purpose of the UB-04 form in medical billing?

   a) To document patient medical history

   b) To submit claims for institutional services

   c) To track patient insurance payments

   d) To schedule patient appointments

62. Which type of modifier is used to indicate a service was provided on a different date than the original service?

   a) -25

   b) -52

   c) -59

   d) -76

63. What is the purpose of a superbill in the billing process?

   a) To track patient appointments

   b) To document services rendered for billing

   c) To collect payments from patients

   d) To manage electronic health records

64. Which ICD-10-CM code is used for a routine check-up?

   a) Z00.00

   b) Z01.419

   c) Z02.0

   d) Z02.1

65. What is the primary purpose of medical coding audits?

a) To evaluate the performance of healthcare providers

b) To ensure compliance and accuracy in coding

c) To prepare for insurance reimbursements

d) To train new coding staff

66. Which organization develops and updates HCPCS Level II codes?

a) American Medical Association (AMA)

b) Centers for Medicare & Medicaid Services (CMS)

c) World Health Organization (WHO)

d) American Health Information Management Association (AHIMA)

67. What does the term "global fee" mean in medical billing?

a) The total charges for a single service

b) A flat fee for all services in a procedure

c) The insurance company's payment limit

d) The amount a patient pays for all services in a year

68. In which situation would you use a "-59" modifier?

a) To indicate a service is bilateral

b) To indicate a distinct procedural service

c) To indicate a professional service only

d) To indicate that a service was repeated

69. What is the role of a medical billing specialist?

   a) To provide patient care directly

   b) To prepare and submit insurance claims

   c) To conduct medical research

   d) To diagnose patient conditions

70. Which code system is primarily used to report surgical procedures?

   a) ICD-10-CM

   b) CPT

   c) HCPCS Level II

   d) CDT

71. What does the modifier "-LT" indicate in medical coding?

   a) The service was provided on the left side of the body

   b) The service was provided on the right side of the body

   c) The procedure was repeated

   d) The service was performed bilaterally

72. Which code is used to report the administration of a COVID-19 vaccine?

   a) CPT

   b) HCPCS Level II

   c) ICD-10-CM

   d) CDT

73. What is a common reason for a claim denial related to coding errors?

   a) Incorrect procedure code

   b) Duplicate services billed

   c) Patient did not show up for the appointment

   d) Patient is out of network

74. Which code is used to report an annual wellness visit in ICD-10-CM?

   a) Z00.00

   b) Z01.419

   c) Z00.121

   d) Z02.1

75. What does a "pre-authorization" requirement mean in medical billing?

   a) Approval from the patient to bill their insurance

   b) Insurance approval before services are rendered

   c) A form that must be signed by the provider

   d) The patient's agreement to pay for all services

76. What type of service is coded with CPT Category III codes?

   a) Established medical procedures

   b) Experimental procedures and emerging technology

   c) Preventive services

   d) Surgical services

77. Which ICD-10-CM category would you use to code for complications of care?

  a) Z codes

  b) T codes

  c) O codes

  d) S codes

78. What is the function of a claims examiner?

  a) To treat patients directly

  b) To review claims for accuracy and compliance

  c) To schedule patient appointments

  d) To provide patient education

79. In medical billing, what does "EOB" stand for?

  a) Explanation of Benefits

  b) End of Bill

  c) Evaluation of Billing

  d) Estimate of Benefits

80. What is the primary purpose of the National Provider Identifier (NPI)?

  a) To track patient diagnoses

  b) To identify healthcare providers

  c) To manage insurance claims

  d) To code medical procedures

81. What is the main purpose of the CMS-1500 form in medical billing?

   a) To submit claims for outpatient services

   b) To record patient medical history

   c) To track insurance reimbursements

   d) To schedule patient appointments

82. Which of the following is a component of the Global Surgical Package?

   a) Preoperative visits

   b) Follow-up visits

   c) Postoperative care

   d) All of the above

83. In medical coding, what does the term "denial" refer to?

   a) The insurance company's refusal to pay a claim

   b) The patient's refusal to pay

   c) A delay in processing a claim

   d) An error in billing

84. Which of the following best describes "medical necessity"?

   a) A service that is required by the patient

   b) A service that is covered by insurance

   c) A service that is appropriate for the diagnosis or treatment

   d) Any service requested by the provider

85. What is the purpose of using a "place of service" code?

   a) To indicate where a service was provided

   b) To track the cost of services

   c) To determine patient eligibility

   d) To classify the type of insurance

86. Which of the following is a feature of the HCPCS Level II coding system?

   a) It includes codes for outpatient services only

   b) It is used primarily for medical procedures

   c) It includes codes for non-physician services and supplies

   d) It is limited to surgical procedures

87. What does the modifier "-51" indicate in CPT coding?

   a) It indicates a repeat procedure

   b) It indicates a bilateral procedure

   c) It indicates multiple procedures

   d) It indicates a professional service only

88. Which organization maintains the Current Procedural Terminology (CPT) codes?

   a) Centers for Medicare & Medicaid Services (CMS)

   b) American Medical Association (AMA)

   c) National Center for Health Statistics (NCHS)

   d) World Health Organization (WHO)

89. What type of service would be classified with an "A" code in HCPCS Level II?

a) Durable medical equipment

b) Anesthesia services

c) Ambulance services

d) Surgical procedures

90. In ICD-10-CM, which character is used as a placeholder?

a) X

b) Z

c) Y

d) W

91. What does the modifier "-50" indicate in medical coding?

a) The service was provided on both sides of the body

b) The service was bilateral

c) The procedure was repeated

d) The service was provided on the left side only

92. Which code would you use to report a new patient office visit in CPT?

a) 99201

b) 99211

c) 99203

d) 99212

93. What is the purpose of a remittance advice (RA)?

   a) To inform the provider about the status of a claim

   b) To schedule patient appointments

   c) To document patient history

   d) To provide coding updates

94. Which of the following codes is used for mental health services in ICD-10-CM?

   a) F codes

   b) G codes

   c) R codes

   d) Z codes

95. What does the term "upcoding" refer to in medical billing?

   a) Billing for a lower level of service than provided

   b) Billing for a higher level of service than provided

   c) Billing for services not rendered

   d) Using outdated codes

96. What is the role of a medical coder in the billing process?

   a) To provide direct patient care

   b) To interpret clinical documentation and assign codes

   c) To handle patient inquiries

d) To manage insurance payments

97. In which situation would a "-22" modifier be used?

  a) When the procedure is more complex than usual

  b) For bilateral procedures

  c) For repeat procedures

  d) For professional services only

98. What is the purpose of a medical billing software system?

  a) To perform patient surgeries

  b) To manage coding updates

  c) To streamline billing and claims processes

  d) To track patient vitals

99. Which part of Medicare primarily covers outpatient services?

  a) Part A

  b) Part B

  c) Part C

  d) Part D

100. What type of code is used to report a patient's allergy to penicillin in ICD-10-CM?

  a) T code

  b) Z code

c) S code

d) E code

ANSWERS

1. **B) ICD-10-CM**

2. **B) Surgical procedures and medical services**

3. **C) World Health Organization (WHO)**

4. **A) Healthcare Common Procedure Coding System**

5. **A) 50**

6. **B) To ensure healthcare providers are paid for services rendered**

7. **C) V codes**

8. **D) HCPCS Level II**

9. **A) Billing for a higher level of service than was provided**

10. **C) 22**

11. **C) Tracking performance measures**

12. **B) Using separate codes for procedures that should be billed together**

13. **B) I10**

14. **C) L**

15. **C) Factors influencing health status and contact with health services**

16. **B) Z code**

17. **A) American Medical Association (AMA)**

18. **B) To ensure accuracy and compliance with coding standards**

19. **A) 21 - Inpatient Hospital**

20. **A) The time frame when all services related to a procedure are included in the original charge**

21. **B) International Classification of Diseases, 10th Revision - Clinical Modification**

22. **B) For experimental and emerging technologies**

23. **A) U**

24. **A) Multiple modifiers are applied**

25. **C) A service that is necessary for the diagnosis or treatment of a patient's condition**

26. **B) S code**

27. **C) Incorrect primary diagnosis order**

28. **B) To provide additional information about a procedure or service**

29. **C) 76**

30. **C) R00-R99**

31. **A) Z codes in ICD-10-CM**

32. **A) Assigning a lower code than what was performed**

33. **A) Duplicate claim**

34. **B) HCPCS Level II**

35. **C) To review and approve or deny insurance claims**

36. **A) ICD-10-PCS**

37. **A) Combining two or more related codes into a single code**

38. **B) Placeholder character**

39. **B) CPT codes**

40. **B) A codes**

41. **B) Coding manual**

42. **A) Category I**

43. **D) American Medical Association (AMA)**

44. **B) -RT**

45. **A) Part A**

46. **C) To document the services provided and their corresponding codes for billing**

47. **B) Billing for services not provided**

48. **C) The insurance company responsible for payment**

49. **B) CPT codes 00100-01999**

50. **A) CMS-1500**

51. **C) Multiple modifiers apply to the code**

52. **B) Deductible**

53. **A) To code inpatient procedures**

54. **A) -26**

55. **C) Service was not justified by patient's diagnosis**

56. **D) CDT**

57. **B) The maximum amount an insurance company will pay for a service**

58. **A) The provider agrees to accept the insurance payment as full payment**

59. **C) HCPCS Level II**

60. **B) The percentage of a service cost shared between patient and insurer**

61. **b) To submit claims for institutional services**

62. d) -76

63. b) To document services rendered for billing

64. a) Z00.00

65. b) To ensure compliance and accuracy in coding

66. b) Centers for Medicare & Medicaid Services (CMS)

67. b) A flat fee for all services in a procedure

68. b) To indicate a distinct procedural service

69. b) To prepare and submit insurance claims

70. b) CPT

71. a) The service was provided on the left side of the body

72. b) HCPCS Level II

73. a) Incorrect procedure code

74. c) Z00.121

75. b) Insurance approval before services are rendered

76. b) Experimental procedures and emerging technology

77. b) T codes

78. b) To review claims for accuracy and compliance

79. a) Explanation of Benefits

80. b) To identify healthcare providers

81. a) To submit claims for outpatient services

82. d) All of the above

83. a) The insurance company's refusal to pay a claim

84. c) A service that is appropriate for the diagnosis or treatment

85. a) To indicate where a service was provided

86. c) It includes codes for non-physician services and supplies

87. c) It indicates multiple procedures

88. b) American Medical Association (AMA)

89. a) Durable medical equipment

90. a) X

91. a) The service was provided on both sides of the body

92. c) 99203

93. a) To inform the provider about the status of a claim

94. a) F codes

95. b) Billing for a higher level of service than provided

96. b) To interpret clinical documentation and assign codes

97. a) When the procedure is more complex than usual

98. c) To streamline billing and claims processes

99. b) Part B

100. b) Z code

Medical Billing and Coding Job Hunting Resources

Navigating the job market can be a challenging endeavor, especially for newcomers to the field of medical billing and coding. However, an abundance of resources are available to streamline your job search and to increase the likelihood of finding a position that matches your skills, interests, and career aspirations. This chapter will provide an in-depth look at various job hunting resources specifically tailored for medical billing and coding professionals.

Online Job Portals for Medical Billing and Coding Jobs

Online job portals have become the go-to source for job seekers in recent years. They provide an efficient platform for professionals to search for jobs that align with their qualifications and interests.

Websites such as Indeed, Glassdoor, and LinkedIn provide vast databases of job postings, including roles in medical billing and coding. When using these platforms, be sure to optimize your job search by using relevant keywords like "Medical Biller," "Medical Coder," "CPC" (Certified Professional Coder), or "CCS" (Certified Coding Specialist). In addition, set up email alerts for these roles to be immediately notified when new jobs are posted.

Specialized healthcare job portals can also provide valuable leads. Websites like Health eCareers, HealthcareJobSite, and MedJobsCafe specifically cater to healthcare professions, increasing the likelihood of finding postings relevant to medical billing and coding.

Recruitment Agencies Specializing in Healthcare

In addition to online job portals, recruitment agencies that specialize in healthcare can be a valuable resource. These agencies work closely with healthcare facilities and private practices, giving them inside knowledge about job openings, some of which may not be advertised publicly.

Companies like AMN Healthcare, HealthCare Support, and Maxim Healthcare Services are among the leading healthcare staffing agencies. Engaging with such agencies can provide personalized guidance in your job search and potentially open doors to a broader range of opportunities.

Social Media Networking for Job Opportunities

Beyond traditional job portals and recruitment agencies, social media platforms can be surprisingly effective for job searching. LinkedIn, for instance, allows you to build a professional network, join groups related to medical billing and coding, and engage with potential employers.

Twitter and Facebook also offer possibilities, with many companies posting job openings on their pages. You can follow healthcare organizations and join groups related to your profession to stay updated on job opportunities. Remember to maintain a professional image on these platforms as potential employers often review these profiles during the hiring process.

Medical Billing and Coding Job Fairs and Hiring Events

Job fairs and hiring events present another avenue to explore job opportunities. These events allow you to interact directly with recruiters and hiring managers, making personal connections that could be beneficial in your job search.

To find these events, regularly check the websites of local healthcare facilities, universities, and job search websites. Professional organizations often host job fairs as well, so keep an eye on their event calendars.

Professional Organizations and Their Job Boards

Professional organizations such as the American Health Information Management Association (AHIMA), the American Academy of Professional Coders (AAPC), and the Healthcare Business Management Association (HBMA) provide numerous resources for medical billing and coding professionals.

These organizations often maintain job boards on their websites, featuring listings from employers specifically seeking the expertise of their members. In addition to job postings, these organizations provide networking events, continuing education resources, and industry news updates, all of which can enhance your job search and career development.

Continuing Education and Certifications for Better Job Prospects

In the rapidly evolving field of healthcare, keeping your skills and knowledge up to date is crucial. Pursuing continuing education and earning additional certifications can dramatically improve your job prospects.

Many professional organizations offer continuing education programs and certifications. For instance, AAPC offers certifications such as the Certified Professional Coder (CPC) and Certified Outpatient Coding (COC), among others.

Likewise, AHIMA offers the Certified Coding Specialist (CCS) and Certified Health Data Analyst (CHDA) credentials. These credentials demonstrate a high level of proficiency and commitment to the field, making you a more attractive candidate to employers.

Remember, landing a job in medical billing and coding is more than just having the required education and certifications. It involves a proactive and strategic job search, leveraging all available resources, and continually improving your skills and knowledge to stay competitive in the field.

Chapter 2: Preparing for Your Job Hunt in Medical Billing and Coding

In the competitive field of medical billing and coding, having the right qualifications is just one piece of the puzzle. To stand out from the crowd, you need a comprehensive strategy that showcases your skills, passion, and professionalism. This chapter will guide you through the key steps of preparing for your job hunt.

Crafting a Winning Resume

A well-crafted resume is your ticket to getting noticed by employers in medical billing and coding. Here are some key points to consider:

- **Clear and Concise Format**: Your resume should be easy to read, with clear headings and bullet points. Start with a strong summary statement, followed by sections on your work experience, education, certifications, and skills.

- **Relevant Work Experience**: Highlight your most relevant work experiences, placing emphasis on your accomplishments rather than just job duties. Use action verbs and quantify achievements where possible, for example, "Improved coding accuracy by 15%".

- **Certifications and Education**: List all relevant certifications such as CPC (Certified Professional Coder), CCS (Certified Coding Specialist), etc. Also, include your educational background, specifically your degree and any specialized training in medical billing and coding.

- **Relevant Skills**: Highlight key skills for medical billing and coding, such as attention to detail, knowledge of medical terminology, proficiency in coding software, and strong communication skills.

Remember to tailor your resume to each job application, echoing the language and requirements stated in the job description.

Building a Strong LinkedIn Profile

LinkedIn is a powerful tool for professionals in any industry, and medical billing and coding is no exception. Here's how to make the most of your profile:

- **Profile Picture and Headline**: Use a professional-looking photo and craft a compelling headline that succinctly showcases your profession and expertise.

- **Summary Section**: Write a concise, engaging summary that encapsulates your career journey, skills, and what you bring to the table.

- **Experience and Education**: List your professional experiences and education similarly to your resume, but feel free to go into more detail and include any projects or initiatives you've contributed to.

- **Skills and Endorsements**: Add relevant skills to your profile and seek endorsements from colleagues and managers to add credibility.

- **Recommendations**: Request recommendations from colleagues, teachers, or managers who can attest to your abilities and professionalism.

Remember to engage with others on the platform by sharing and commenting on relevant content, joining groups related to medical billing and coding, and connecting with professionals in the field.

Developing a Portfolio that Stands Out

A portfolio can be a fantastic way to demonstrate your competence and passion for medical billing and coding. Here's how to create one:

- **Case Studies**: Showcasing your real-world experience with anonymized case studies is an excellent way to demonstrate your expertise and problem-solving skills. Explain how you resolved challenging billing issues, or how your coding improved a practice's revenue cycle.

- **Certifications**: A portfolio offers the opportunity to provide more detail about your certifications. Consider discussing what you learned, key projects, and how you have applied these learnings in the workplace.

- **Continued Learning**: Show your dedication to your profession by documenting your continued learning journey. Discuss conferences you've attended, webinars you found useful, or additional courses you're taking.

You can build your portfolio using a variety of online platforms or create a simple PDF document that you can email to prospective employers.

Networking Strategies in the Healthcare Industry

Networking is a key part of any job search strategy. Here are some ways to effectively network in the healthcare industry:

- **Professional Organizations**: Joining organizations like the AAPC (American Academy of Professional Coders) or AHIMA (American Health Information Management Association) can provide opportunities to meet like-minded professionals and learn about unadvertised job openings.

- **Industry Events**: Attending industry events, whether in-person or virtual, can help you connect with industry professionals and potential employers.

- **Alumni Networks**: Leverage your college or training program's alumni network. Fellow alumni often have valuable insights and connections in the industry.

- **Informational Interviews**: Request informational interviews with professionals in the field. This is a great way to learn more about different roles and companies in the industry.

In conclusion, a successful job hunt in medical billing and coding requires a blend of a well-crafted resume, a strong online presence, a demonstrable portfolio, and effective networking strategies. The preparation may seem extensive, but remember: the more effort you put into these stages, the greater your chances are of landing your ideal job.

Chapter 3: The Interview Guide for Medical Billing and Coding

Navigating an interview can be a daunting task, particularly in the specialized field of medical billing and coding. Knowing what to expect and how to prepare can significantly boost your confidence and performance. This chapter serves as a comprehensive guide for acing medical billing and coding interviews.

Understanding the Interview Process

The interview process for medical billing and coding jobs usually follows a typical structure: a phone screening, a first round interview (often conducted via video call), and a final interview (usually in-person).

During the phone screening, the recruiter verifies your basic qualifications and checks if you're a good fit for the job on a fundamental level. In the first round interview, you'll likely meet with a hiring manager or supervisor who will delve deeper into your professional background and technical skills. The final round may involve meeting with senior team members or other stakeholders. At this stage, your cultural fit with the team and company are often assessed.

Understanding this process can help you anticipate what each stage will entail, allowing you to better prepare and succeed.

Typical Medical Billing and Coding Interview Questions and Answers

Knowing what questions to expect can give you an edge during the interview. Here are some common questions and how you might approach them:

- **What coding systems are you familiar with?** *Your Answer:* "I am proficient in ICD-10, CPT, and HCPCS Level II coding systems. During my time at XYZ Healthcare, I used these coding systems daily to ensure accurate and efficient medical billing."

- **Can you describe a challenging billing situation and how you resolved it?** *Your Answer:* "At my previous job, I encountered a situation where an insurance company repeatedly denied a claim due to a coding error. I meticulously reviewed the patient's records, identified the mistake, and corrected the codes. I then resubmitted the claim, which was approved. This experience emphasized the importance of attention to detail in coding."

Remember to provide specific examples from your experience when answering these questions.

Technical Skills Evaluation During Interviews

As a medical biller and coder, your technical skills will be a crucial focus during interviews. You may be asked questions about medical terminology, coding systems, insurance procedures, and the use of billing software.

In some cases, employers may administer a coding test to assess your competency. It's important to stay updated on the latest coding practices and software to excel in this part of the interview.

Soft Skills and Their Importance in Interviews

Though technical skills are crucial, don't underestimate the importance of soft skills in medical billing and coding. These include communication skills, attention to detail, organizational skills, problem-solving, and the ability to work under pressure.

You can showcase these skills by using examples from your past experience during the interview. For instance, you might share a story about a time when your strong organizational skills enabled you to manage a high volume of claims effectively.

Dressing for Success: What to Wear to Interviews

How you present yourself at an interview is a direct reflection of your professionalism. For medical billing and coding interviews, business or business-casual attire is generally appropriate. For men, this could mean dress slacks and a collared shirt; for women, a dress, skirt or slacks paired with a blouse works well. It's always better to be slightly overdressed than underdressed.

Regardless of your outfit choice, ensure your clothes are clean, ironed, and well-fitting. Keep jewelry and makeup minimal and opt for professional-looking footwear.

Post-interview Follow-ups and Thank-you Notes

The interview process doesn't end when you walk out the door. Following up with a thank-you note is a courteous way to express your appreciation for the interviewer's time. It also reinforces your interest in the role and keeps you fresh in the interviewer's mind.

In your note, thank the interviewer for their time, express your continued interest in the role, and reiterate how you can contribute to the team. Email is a perfectly acceptable medium for a thank-you note, and it's best to send it within 24 hours of your interview.

Chapter 4: Advancing Your Career in Medical Billing and Coding

Climbing the ladder in medical billing and coding requires dedication, strategic planning, and a commitment to lifelong learning. In this chapter, we explore how to continue growing and advancing in your career while maintaining a healthy work-life balance.

Continuing Education Opportunities

Continuing education is essential to stay abreast of changes in healthcare laws, insurance policies, and coding practices. Here are some opportunities to consider:

- **Online Courses and Webinars**: Numerous platforms offer online courses and webinars focused on medical coding, billing, healthcare regulations, and more. These offer flexible learning opportunities that can fit into your schedule.

- **Industry Conferences**: Conferences such as the AAPC's HEALTHCON or AHIMA's annual conference provide excellent opportunities to learn from industry leaders, network with peers, and stay updated on industry trends and changes.

- **Training Programs**: Many employers offer in-house training programs. Taking advantage of these programs can help you stay up-to-date, enhance your skills, and demonstrate your commitment to your career.

Relevant Certifications to Pursue

Obtaining advanced certifications can bolster your expertise and credibility, making you more competitive in the job market. Here are a few worth considering:

- **Certified Professional Coder (CPC)**: If not already earned, this is a fundamental certification for anyone in medical coding.

- **Certified Professional Medical Auditor (CPMA)**: This certification reflects expertise in medical auditing, a valuable skill for identifying problematic coding and billing patterns.

- **Certified Risk Adjustment Coder (CRC)**: This certification is focused on risk adjustment coding, which is increasingly important in ensuring accurate patient care data.

- **Certified Documentation Expert Outpatient (CDEO)**: This certification demonstrates expertise in reviewing outpatient documentation for accuracy to secure quality patient care and optimal reimbursement.

Remember that each certification requires ongoing education to maintain, ensuring that certified professionals stay current in their field.

Industry Trends to Keep an Eye On

Keeping up with industry trends allows you to adapt and grow with the field. Notable trends include:

- **Automation and AI**: Automated systems and artificial intelligence are increasingly being used to streamline billing and coding processes. Familiarity with these technologies can be a significant asset.

- **Telemedicine**: The rise of telemedicine has brought changes to coding and billing practices. Understanding the specific codes and billing procedures for telemedicine is essential.

- **Changes in Laws and Regulations**: Healthcare regulations and insurance laws are always evolving. Staying informed about these changes is crucial to ensure accurate and compliant coding and billing.

Maintaining Work-Life Balance in the Medical Billing and Coding Field

While advancing your career, it's also important to maintain a healthy work-life balance. Here are some tips:

- **Set Boundaries**: Try to keep your work and personal life separate. Set specific work hours and stick to them as much as possible.

- **Take Breaks**: Regular breaks can help prevent burnout. Try to step away from your work station every couple of hours, even if it's just for a few minutes.

- **Stay Active**: Physical activity can help reduce stress and improve mental health. Incorporate exercise into your routine, whether it's a daily walk or a workout at the gym.

- **Practice Mindfulness**: Techniques such as meditation, deep breathing, and yoga can help maintain mental wellness, reduce stress, and improve focus.

In summary, advancing your career in medical billing and coding involves continuous education, pursuing relevant certifications, keeping abreast of industry trends, and maintaining a healthy work-life balance. With the right strategy, you can enjoy a fulfilling and successful career in this dynamic field.

Chapter 5: Conclusion

The Future of Medical Billing and Coding Jobs

The field of medical billing and coding holds an exciting and promising future. It is continually evolving in response to technological advancements, regulatory changes, and shifts in healthcare delivery, making it a dynamic and rewarding career choice.

Advancements in automation and artificial intelligence have the potential to streamline many aspects of medical coding and billing, improving efficiency and accuracy. This doesn't mean that machines will replace human coders and billers; rather, professionals in the field will be working in tandem with these technologies, leveraging them to enhance their performance. As such, staying tech-savvy and embracing new technological tools will be key for future success.

The growth of telemedicine and other digital health services is also reshaping the landscape. These changes bring unique coding and billing challenges that require updated knowledge and skills.

Given these trends, it is clear that the demand for competent, well-trained medical billing and coding professionals will continue to grow. As such, individuals in this field can look forward to a stable career with abundant opportunities for learning and advancement.

Final Words of Advice for Aspiring Medical Billers and Coders

If you're starting your journey in medical billing and coding, remember that success in this field requires continuous learning and adaptation. Embrace the opportunity to learn, whether it's through formal education, on-the-job training, professional certifications, or industry events. Staying current with industry trends, regulations, and technologies is crucial.

Keep honing both your technical and soft skills. While coding and billing skills are essential, soft skills like communication, problem-solving, and attention to detail are equally important and can set you apart.

Lastly, cultivate a strong professional network. Join professional organizations, attend industry conferences, and leverage social media platforms like LinkedIn. Networking can open up new opportunities, provide learning experiences, and offer invaluable support throughout your career journey.

Appendix: Resources and Links

The following resources can help you kick-start or advance your career in medical billing and coding:

- **American Academy of Professional Coders (AAPC)**: Provides certification programs, continuing education, networking opportunities, and industry updates.

- **American Health Information Management Association (AHIMA)**: Offers various certifications, training programs, and a wealth of resources for health information management professionals.

- **Healthcare Business Management Association (HBMA)**: Provides resources, advocacy, education, and certification for professionals in healthcare revenue cycle management.

- **LinkedIn Groups**: Groups such as 'Medical Billing and Coding Forum' and 'Medical Billers and Coders' are great platforms to connect with other professionals, ask questions, and share insights.